Praise for
CONCUSSION RESCU

"The definitive guide to treating traumatic brain injury (TBI), from mild to severe, *Concussion Rescue* provides the most up-to-date effective strategies for recovering your health and your life. Dr. Chapek has created an essential resource for anyone struggling with the effects of concussion."

—**Mark Hyman, MD,** #1 *New York Times* bestselling
    author and director, Cleveland Clinic Center
    for Functional Medicine

"I so wish this outstanding book had been available when my son had a soccer concussion in high school. It took six months before he was back to normal. He could have recovered much more quickly if we had known of Dr. Chapek's protocols. Every parent with active children must read this book to be prepared for the inevitable.

—**Joseph Pizzorno, ND**, Founding President,
    Bastyr University

"A comprehensive natural program that addresses the underlying neurophysiology of the effects of concussions and traumatic brain injuries. Easy to read and packed full of practical, clinically relevant information. The well thought out program in *Concussion Rescue* will dramatically improve our current 'wait and rest' medical model for concussions and traumatic brain injuries."

—**James M. Greenblatt, MD,** chief medical officer,
    Walden Behavioral Care, medical director,
    Psychiatry Redefined

"Finally, a breakthrough against the brain injury epidemic! Dr. Chapek skillfully explains how to use SPECT functional brain mapping, cognitive testing, and meticulous lab work, along with concentrated oxygen, diet, supplements, and numerous other nontoxic treatments, to rescue the brain from TBI. Anyone who wants their brain to work better will benefit from reading this book."

—**Parris M. Kidd, PhD,** University of California, Berkeley, brain nutraceutical pioneer

"In *Concussion Rescue*, Dr. Chapek lays out in detail exactly what you need to know in order to recover from a traumatic brain injury (TBI) or concussion. Never before has anyone created a 'TBI first aid kit,' which includes basic nutrients and supplements to take immediately after injury to reduce inflammation and cell death to help *prevent* many of the insidious post-TBI symptoms that plague so many people."

—**Drew Sinatra, ND,** Lac Integrative Medicine

"*Concussion Rescue* is an excellent guide, reference, and road map to understanding and recovering from brain injury. Dr Chapek eloquently provides a detailed tool kit and action plan to assist in repairing the brain. I will read *Concussion Rescue* and refer to it again and again."

—**Adam Rinde, ND**

CONCUSSION RESCUE

A Comprehensive Program to Heal Traumatic Brain Injury

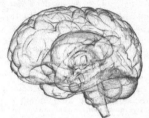

DR. KABRAN CHAPEK

Foreword by
DANIEL AMEN, MD

CITADEL PRESS
Kensington Publishing Corp.
www.kensingtonbooks.com

CITADEL PRESS BOOKS are published by
Kensington Publishing Corp.
119 West 40th Street
New York, NY 10018

All images, unless otherwise noted, are courtesy The Amen Clinic.

PUBLISHER'S NOTE
The information presented in this book is the result of years of practice experience and
research by the author. The information in this book, by necessity, is of a general nature
and is not a substitute for an evaluation and/or treatment by a competent medical special-
ist. If you believe you or a family member might have a brain injury and/or are in need of
medical intervention, please see a medical practitioner or go the nearest emergency room
immediately. This book is not a replacement for the medical assessment and treatment of a
brain injury, including a concussion. Please see a medical practitioner or go to the nearest
emergency room as soon as possible. The stories in this book are based on true events. The
names and circumstances of the stories have been changed to protect the anonymity and
privacy of patients.

All Kensington titles, imprints, and distributed lines are available at special quantity dis-
counts for bulk purchases for sales promotions, premiums, fund-raising, educational, or
institutional use. Special book excerpts or customized printings can also be created to
fit specific needs. For details, write or phone the office of the Kensington sales manager:
Kensington Publishing Corp., 119 West 40th Street, New York, NY 10018, attn: Sales
Department; phone 1-800-221-2647.

ISBN-13: 978-0-8065-4023-8
ISBN-10: 0-8065-4023-0

First trade paperback printing: February 2020

10 9 8 7 6 5 4 3 2 1

Printed in the United States of America

Electronic edition: February 2020

ISBN-13: 978-0-8065-4024-5 (e-book)
ISBN-10: 0-8065-4024-9 (e-book)

To my lovely, wise, and supportive wife, Drie.
To my wonderful children, whose brains I cherish.
To my parents, who taught me about health.

CONTENTS

Contents

FOREWORD
by Daniel Amen

Your brain is at the core of what makes you who you are. When it works right, you work right; when it is troubled for whatever reason, you are much more likely to have trouble in your life. Many people think the brain is rubbery and fixed within the skull, but it isn't. Your brain is soft, about the consistency of soft butter, tofu, or custard—somewhere between egg whites and gelatin. It floats in cerebrospinal fluid and is housed in a very hard skull that has many sharp bony ridges (see illustration on next page). As such, it is easily damaged.

Whiplash, jarring motions (think Shaken Baby Syndrome), blast injuries, and blows to the head can cause the brain to slosh around, slamming into the hard interior ridges of the skull. There are several mechanisms of physical brain trauma:

- Bruising
- Broken blood vessels and bleeding
- Increased pressure
- Lack of oxygen
- Damage to nerve cell connections
- Spilling out of tau proteins, which cause inflammatory reactions, from brain cells that have been ripped open

In addition, because your pituitary gland (master hormone regulator) sits in a vulnerable part of your skull, it is often damaged in head injuries, causing significant hormonal imbalances.

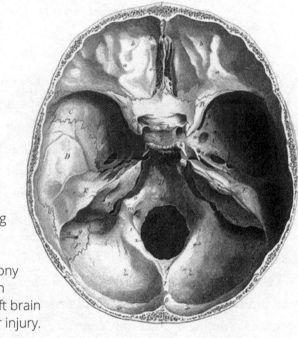

A Look Inside the Skull. Looking down from the top, you can see the protective bony ridges, which can damage your soft brain in an accident or injury.

According to the CDC, there are over two million new head injuries in the US every year. That means over the last forty years, more than 80 million people have sustained head injuries. And the number of concussions is also rising, especially among children. From 2010 to 2015, concussion diagnoses jumped 43 percent among the general population. For young people 10 to 19 years of age, however, concussion diagnoses skyrocketed 71 percent. We have to do a much better job of preventing TBIs and repairing the brain when they occur.

Common causes of head injuries include:

- **Falls:** falling out of bed, down steps, off ladders; slipping in the bath or shower.

- **Motor vehicle collisions** involving cars, motorcycles, or bicycles, as well as pedestrians.

- **Violence:** gunshot wounds, assaults, domestic violence, or child abuse.

- **Sports injuries:** in addition to football, they are common in soccer, boxing, baseball, lacrosse, skateboarding, hockey, cycling, basketball, and other high-impact or extreme sports.

- **Explosive blasts** and other combat injuries.

At Amen Clinics, we see patients with head injuries from all of these causes. In particular, we have been studying the association between football and brain injuries for three decades. When I first started looking at SPECT scans in 1991, I saw Pop Warner and high school players between the ages of 8 and 18 with clear evidence of traumatic brain injuries. I was horrified. And then I saw college players whose brains showed even more damage. In the past decade, I've met with over 300 active and former NFL players whose scans were even worse. Yet, using the Amen Clinics' BRIGHT MINDS program, described in this book, 80 percent of our players show improvements in blood flow, mood, memory, and sleep.

At the time of this writing, more than 350,000 military veterans have sustained a TBI since the year 2000. This means the Iraq and Afghanistan wars will likely have a 70-year tail, as these veterans will have an increased risk for psychiatric issues and dementia. The impact of those TBIs will spread beyond the veterans themselves and affect their children and succeeding generations.

Research shows that head injuries increase the risk of:

- Depression
- Anxiety and panic disorders
- Psychosis
- PTSD
- Suicide
- Drug and alcohol abuse
- ADHD
- Learning problems
- Borderline and antisocial personality disorders
- Dementia
- Aggression
- Homelessness
- Victimization
- Loss of or changes in sense of smell or taste

Head trauma may also increase the risk of incarceration. In the US, 25 to 87 percent of inmates say they have suffered a TBI compared with 25 to 38 percent in the general population. And the latest statistics from the Bureau of Justice Statistics show that 181,500 veterans are incarcerated.

In our database of tens of thousands of patients, 40 percent had a significant brain injury before they came to see us. When people ask me what is the single most important lesson I've learned from looking at over 170,000 brain scans, I reply, "Mild traumatic brain injury is a major cause of psychiatric problems, and very few people know it."

I actually hate the word "mild" applied to traumatic brain injuries or concussions, because it implies that they didn't cause lasting damage, which is often not the case. Anyone who has played a contact sport has likely also experienced many sub-concussive blows, where the brain was jostled but did not cause immediate symptoms.

It is important to note that many people forget they've had a significant head injury in the past. At Amen Clinics, we routinely ask patients several times whether or not they have had a head injury. Our intake paperwork asks the question "Have you ever had a head injury?" The historian, who gathers patients' histories before they see the physician, asks them again about head injuries. The computer testing we have patients complete asks a third time about head injuries. If I see *no, no, no* to the question of head injuries, I'll ask again. If I get a fourth no, I will then say, "Are you sure? Have you ever fallen out of a tree, fallen off a fence, or dove into a shallow pool? Did you play contact sports? Have you ever been in a car accident?"

I'm constantly amazed at how many people think their head injuries were too insignificant to mention. For others, they simply do not remember the incident, as amnesia is a common occurrence in head traumas. When asked the question for the fifth time, one patient put his hand on his forehead and said, "Oh yeah! When I was 5 years old, I fell out of a second-story window." Likewise, I have had other patients forget they went through windshields, fell out of moving vehicles, or were knocked unconscious when they fell off their bicycles.

Concussion Rescue is written by a smart, deeply caring naturopathic physician who has worked at Amen Clinics for many years. In the pages of this book you will find hope, help, and a specific plan to improve your brain and rescue your mind.

DANIEL G. AMEN, MD, is the founder of Amen Clinics and the author of *The End of Mental Illness: How Neuroscience Is Transforming Psychiatry and Helping to Prevent or Reverse Anxiety, Depression, Bipolar Disorder, ADHD, Addictions, PTSD, Psychosis, and More.*

A NOTE TO THE READER

I didn't plan or decide early in my career as a naturopathic physician to focus on individuals with brain injuries or brain disorders. When I first started working in mental health, however, I realized this was something I would be doing for the rest of my life because I loved helping people become their most effective selves. Working with patients who have brain problems is extremely fulfilling, because helping someone improve the health of their brain changes their life *right now* and for many years to come.

I have always had a passion for helping my friends and family members feel their best by taking care of their bodies. This was part of my inspiration for studying natural medicine at Bastyr University, a world-renowned school for naturopathic medicine in Seattle, Washington. In fact, Bastyr is what brought me and my wife, Drie, to the Pacific Northwest. We hoped to build our lives in an area that fit with our values of natural health care and our mutual love of the outdoors.

Working at a treatment center in nearby Edmonds, I helped people with severe depression, anxiety, eating disorders, and chemical dependency. Many of the depressed patients had recently been in a psychiatric inpatient unit for a suicide attempt and this was their first step down to a less comprehensive level of care. For others, this was the first help they had found, sometimes after struggling for years on their own. The treatment center's mission was to have naturopathic physicians as the primary doctors, working with a team of other providers to take care of these patients. I developed a deep respect for the highly trained therapists, counselors, and dietitians on staff, and I worked closely with psychiatrists to provide whole-person care.

Through watching patients struggle with depression, anxiety, guilt, and suicidal thoughts, I learned many difficult and wonderful lessons about how the brain works. I treated thousands of patients using nutritional interventions and saw amazing improvements with simple methods. In addition, I learned when medications are needed and can be lifesaving. I saw patients' physical health improve, which in turn helped to lift their depression or help with behavioral or chemical addictions. Eventually, I became the medical director of this facility. I'm grateful for my time there and my training in psychiatry.

My passion for psychiatry and natural medicine was ignited anew when I was asked to join the team at the Amen Clinics Northwest. Dr. Daniel Amen is changing the way psychiatry is practiced, and the model at the Amen Clinics fits exactly with my ideal of providing holistic psychiatric care to patients. I love both the cutting-edge research that we are doing and being able to help patients in our eight clinics across the country. The integrative and progressive approaches we use are grounded in scientific evidence, which is important when it comes to something as challenging as brain problems.

We are always looking for the best ways to help our patients, and I hope this book is one that parents, family members, caregivers, and healthcare providers can use to help those suffering with a traumatic brain injury.

How to Use *Concussion Rescue*

A *concussion* is a form of mild *TBI* (traumatic brain injury). Therefore, I am going to use the terms concussion and TBI interchangeably throughout the book. The same treatments and approach apply whether you are seeking help for a mild or more severe brain injury.

Some of you are coming to this book because you have had a brain injury and haven't been able to heal, or a loved one has had that experience. Others may have had a brain health problem such as depression, anxiety, rage, attention difficulties, fatigue, or memory issues and come to suspect that a past brain injury was the cause of your problems. Either way, this book will provide options for assessment and treatment.

The information in this book is designed to be an adjunct to conventional medical care, not a replacement for it. Your healthcare provider can be one of your greatest assets in your journey to healing. For example, your provider may be able to order and help interpret the critical lab tests in the assessment phase of your program.

Feel free to dive into this book at whatever chapter addresses your issue. For example if you have just had a concussion, you may want to go straight to chapter 5, "First Aid for Your Brain," to find which specific nutrients can help right after such an injury. If you have chronic insomnia, you may want to start with chapter 10 for some help getting a good night's rest; if you are considering hyperbaric oxygen, you might want to skip right to chapter 12.

Whether you are a parent or a coach, have recently had a fall or are a veteran struggling with the aftereffects of a past brain injury, I hope this manual guides you back to health.

1

BACK TO THE DRAWING BOARD

Kevin was an energetic high school soccer player who rev-
eled in every game and practice, a fierce competitor who
broke up offensive attacks with aggressive sliding tackles on
the field.

During a corner kick late in a scoreless game, Kevin posi-
tioned himself just outside the penalty box, knowing that his
teammate would try to "bend it like Beckham" and give him
a chance to headbutt the flying sphere into the back of the net.
The corner kick came in high and fast, and a scrum of players
from both teams converged on the ball.

As Kevin leaped high for a header, his head collided with
another player's skull. There was a sickening *thud,* and the
youngster tumbled to the ground, where he cried out in pain.

Play stopped after the goalie collected the ball, and a half
dozen players from both teams gathered around Kevin. He
wasn't knocked unconscious, but as he pulled himself to his
feet, he was woozy. He was led off the field, where his concerned parents were waiting. When Kevin failed to shake

the cobwebs out of his head, his father and mother rushed him to the emergency room.

Following a long wait, a short examination, and a quick visit to the CT scanner, the ER doc informed Kevin and his parents that he would be "just fine," based on the results of the CT scan. Kevin had suffered a concussion, the doctor said, explaining that a concussion was a form of mild traumatic brain injury—or TBI. Kevin and his parents were told that he should feel back to his old self in a few days or a few weeks, depending on the severity of the concussion. He was directed to "watch and wait and take Tylenol for a headache," which is standard protocol in the traditional medicine world.

Instead of quickly recovering, as most teen boys do, Kevin experienced splitting headaches over the next few weeks that stretched into months. His headaches throbbed so much that he couldn't read more than a few lines of his textbooks at a time. When he fell further and further behind in his schoolwork, Kevin had to withdraw from school. Kevin ended up missing classes for several months because of his symptoms and became very depressed.

Kevin's mom grew increasingly concerned and scheduled an appointment with me at the Amen Clinics in Bellevue, Washington. As a naturopathic doctor (ND), I had been seeing more and more post-concussion patients in recent years as parents sought treatment for their children who were not recovering from mild traumatic injuries. They hoped a more natural or alternative approach would be more effective.

As a doctor of naturopathic medicine, my goal is to treat

the cause and heal the injury versus just recommending over-the-counter pain relievers and rest. Conventional doctors willingly admit that their medical bag is nearly empty when it comes to effective treatment options for mild traumatic brain injuries. However, as you can see, there is nothing mild about Kevin's situation.

My first interview with Kevin did not go well for the young man. When I asked him to describe certain events from the previous day, his responses seemed slow and he had great difficulty remembering even simple things, like what he ate for breakfast. After putting him through a battery of tests and baseline cognitive testing, I immediately started Kevin on a treatment plan consisting of targeted nutrients. I prescribed a formula, based on research, consisting of specific amino acids, vitamins, and minerals shown to be helpful at improving healing from brain injury. I also recommended significant changes to his diet. When Kevin's brain received the correct resources, he was able to move from a dysfunctional idling state into a more functional one within days. As Kevin's headaches diminished, he began to regain his memory. Two weeks later, he was back in school and feeling much better about life.

On his next visit, he asked me a hard question: "Will I be able to play soccer again?"

"I wouldn't want to roll the dice with your brain and your future, but the choice is ultimately up to you," I responded. To play soccer at the competitive level that he was used to playing, I said, would mean risking another concussion and therefore permanent brain injury.

Kevin nodded to signal that he understood, but I could tell he was processing what this meant to his days of playing a sport he loved. Although it took him several weeks to get used to the idea, Kevin ultimately realized that he had gifts other than soccer. He decided to focus on academics and try playing noncontact sports in the future.

Concussions like the one Kevin suffered are all too common. The number of brain injuries sustained each year is in the millions and continues to grow. According to the Centers for Disease Control and Prevention (CDC), there were more than 2.5 million emergency room visits for a variety of brain injuries in 2010, the most recent year available for this vital research. A majority of those brain-related ER visits were from falls, unintentional blunt trauma (such as being hit by an object), vehicular accidents, and injuries suffered on the playing field. These days, it's estimated that 10 percent of athletes will experience a concussion during their season, according to the Sports Concussion Institute.

Unfortunately, countless traumatic brain injuries go undiagnosed because many are brushed off as "just a hit to the head," similar to what Kevin experienced. But thanks to increased media attention, like the movie *Concussion*, starring Will Smith as Dr. Bennet Omalu, the forensic pathologist credited with being the first to discover chronic traumatic encephalopathy (CTE), concussions are being taken more seriously. The word is getting out that repeated hits to the head and ensuing concussions cause long-term brain damage.

The identification of the problem is only half the battle, however. Although advances have been made in emergency neurosurgery, which has helped save thousands of lives, it's well known among brain-injury researchers that we don't have effective treatments for brain injury. In fact, nearly all of the over thirty large-scale trials in this field over the past thirty years have failed to find an effective drug treatment for acute brain injury.

I believe the rising problem of traumatic brain injuries isn't being approached correctly, which is why it's time to go back to the drawing board. I'm not proposing that we start all over, but I feel we need to think differently about the way we approach brain injuries. We can start by looking at what happens with each individual brain injury and match each one with the right treatments.

At Amen Clinics we have a way of remembering to look at concussions in a comprehensive way using the mnemonic BRIGHT MINDS. Each letter stands for a different component that must be considered in order to have the best chance of healing from head injuries. In each chapter I will highlight the BRIGHT MINDS principles that are key to focus on in order to recover from a brain injury.

B—Blood flow: After a hit to the head, blood vessels can be damaged, leading to decreased blood flow. This must be addressed as a core piece of healing from brain injuries. Also lack of exercise (less than twice a week) contributes to deficient blood flow and is a barrier to healing.

R—Retirement/aging: According to the CDC (Centers for Disease Control), visits to the emergency room for TBI-related falls is highest among children ages 0–4 and adults 65 years old and older. The brain may be more vulnerable to the consequences of brain injury when the brain is first developing and when it is older and there is less brain reserve and hormones are at lower levels.

I—Inflammation: Brain injury involves an inflammatory cascade that occurs minutes to hours after a fall or an accident and smolders like a campfire that can last for months and even years. This inflammation is related to chronic symptoms of brain injury. Signs of inflammation can be measured as C-reactive protein and homocysteine in the blood (lab tests will be discussed in chapter 3).

G—Genetics: People with the APOE4 gene have a higher risk of having chronic symptoms after a hit to the head perhaps because individuals with the APOE4 allele may have a greater inflammatory response in general.[1,2]

H—Head trauma: A history of head injuries with or without a loss of consciousness can cause long-term problems and mental illness. Even playing contact sports without having concussions can cause damage to the brain, and the damage is cumulative.

T—Toxins: Alcohol or drug abuse, exposure to toxins in the environment (mold, pollution) or from personal products, and cancer chemotherapy can all worsen brain function and make it harder to heal from brain injury.

M—Mental health: Brain injuries are a significant cause of mental illness. Brain injuries are not considered (most of the time) as a cause of mental illness, however, studies have shown that TBI can cause attentional problems, depression, anxiety, and even psychosis.[3,4,5]

I—Immunity/Infections: Damage to the brain can cause problems with the gut and digestion, creating an environment where food sensitivities can begin and lowering immune function, thus making the body susceptible to a chronic infection like Lyme or Epstein-Barr Virus (EBV).

N—Neurohormone deficiencies: Minor hits to the head can cause full or partial damage to the pituitary gland, causing hormonal deficiencies that may be the cause of some post–concussive syndrome symptoms, such as depression, fatigue, insomnia, low motivation, and attentional and memory problems.

D—Diabesity: Having a diet higher in refined carbohydrates and sugars will put you at higher risk of not recovering from a hit to the head and makes it more likely you will have chronic symptoms after a brain injury. The brain needs the right kinds of fuel to recover and function optimally.

S—Sleep: Brain injuries cause insomnia in a majority of patients who have a concussion, and this is one of the most important aspects to correct if healing is to occur.

A large part of the problem in adequately treating brain injury is that the effects of brain injury are often not immediately evident. Here's an example: Dave, another patient of mine, enjoyed going out and drinking on the weekends. One night after leaving a craft brewery, he was jumped by a couple of guys waiting for him in the parking lot. It seems that the girlfriend of one of the guys had been two-timing him with Dave. This guy and his buddy assaulted Dave with baseball bats and smashed his skull in. He was rushed to a

Seattle hospital that was world-renowned for brain injury and underwent emergency surgery.

During the first month of recuperation, Dave appeared to be coming out of the woods, and before discharge he scored well within the normal range on all of his cognitive testing. However, three months after the violent beatdown, he began to have severe cognitive difficulties. This delayed onset of symptoms, which is actually quite common, catches people off guard since they do not suspect that their memory troubles stem from injuries sustained months or even years earlier. This explains why many are perplexed about why they are experiencing unexplained depression, fatigue, memory problems, dizziness, and headaches.

This was exactly what happened to Dave. A good half a year after his injury, Dave couldn't hold on to his job, had difficulty speaking, and could not focus or concentrate for more than a few minutes at a time. He also acquired a rage problem, often exploding at the slightest perceived offense.

We used to think that if symptoms or lack of function exist for more than a year after a brain injury, then it's highly unlikely there will be any further recovery. Fortunately, evidence is showing that with the proper protocol, significant improvements can be made. In Dave's case, we were able to raise his level of function and lower his anger enough to allow him to return to work on a part-time basis. Dave may continue to improve with further intervention, but there will be a point at which no further gains can be made. However, when it comes to your brain, we should try several different approaches, because your brain is just too important not to have it function optimally. Not every patient will improve as much as Dave, however. Some will improve more, some less, but the good news is that an improved outcome is possible. I have seen time and again that even years after their injuries, patients can recover significant pieces of brain function.

Damage Control

What happens to the brain after a traumatic brain injury, mild or otherwise?

We don't know as much as we would like, but modern science agrees that a direct blow to the head causes neurons and blood vessels to stretch and tear, producing anywhere from mild to severe damage.

What's interesting to me is what happens to the brain *after* the initial damage occurs. In most cases, a cascade of inflammatory chemicals, called cytokines, produces a release of excitatory neurotransmitters and an imbalance of amino acids. Other side effects are cerebral edema (swelling), a lack of nutrition to brain cells, inflammation, and decreased blood supply.

These same mechanisms of damage occur whether the TBI incident is mild or severe. The extent of that damage is typically worse and more apparent in severe traumatic brain injury, where there is typically more swelling. That's not to discount damage from a mild TBI event, which can cause a host of problems. What I hadn't realized until I began working at the Amen Clinics is that *every* brain injury matters, large and small, and that brain injuries are a major source of psychiatric illness (even though the greater medical

9

community has largely dismissed the link between TBI and mental illness).

A brain injury is different for every person, because the mechanism of brain injury is complicated and damage occurs not just at the site of injury. Therefore, treatments should have a similarly multifaceted mechanism of action. The beauty of natural treatments is that they contain hundreds of chemicals acting on many pathways simultaneously to calm the brain and begin the healing process.

Many of the more successful treatments used in clinical trials have focused on reducing death rates by addressing primary damage. One of the treatments is *craniectomy*, which is removing a piece of the skull to decrease pressure. Another is *hypothermia*, which is lowering the patient's body temperature to cool down the brain and decrease swelling and inflammation—the equivalent of putting ice on a sprained ankle or bruised muscle. These treatments of primary injury have reduced the mortality rate and are nothing short of miraculous. In fact, the death rate from brain injury has decreased over the past thirty years from 40–50 percent down to 20–30 percent.[6]

At Stanford University, an undergraduate named Theodore Roth was part of a research project using an intracranial microscope to capture never-before-seen footage of what happens inside the brain minutes to hours after a traumatic blow to the head. The team implanted the microscope in mice's skulls. The mice were then struck on the head, and the internal results were recorded on the microscope.

In his team's model of brain injury, Roth showed how highly

unstable molecules wreak havoc and kill cells all around them. Oxidative damage—basically, rust—also occurs. So, among other troubles, you can picture an injured brain as "rusting out" from the inside.

This is what generally happens to the brain during traumatic injury: tissues are torn, cells are damaged and turn "rusty," and the brain lacks the energy it needs to heal. Inflammation of the tissues around the brain always occurs.

So how does the brain recover—or cope?

In naturopathic medical school, we learned that inflammation has three hallmark signs: redness, pain, and swelling. Imagine a sprained ankle. The lower leg is swollen with fluid, red, and sore to the touch. Through these reactions, the body is protecting the injured ankle. We may apply ice and elevate the leg to reduce these symptoms.

The brain, however, does not necessarily "appear" hurt, which is why many believe they're going to be all right. The injury can't be seen; we don't see the swelling or feel the inflammation and heat associated with traumatic brain injury. And the brain is difficult to cool because the excess fluid doesn't have anyplace to go. When that happens, the excess fluid harms brain tissue simply due to the increased pressure it causes. The brain swelling can be gradual, which is why symptoms may not show up until weeks after injury.

Earlier I said that the key is to look at what happens with each individual brain injury and match each one with the correct treatments. What I love about the Stanford study is that the researchers did that. They saw oxidative damage and applied the antioxidant glutathione topically on the skin, which then passed right through the skull into the brain.

Glutathione is the body's premier antioxidant and is produced naturally by the brain, liver, and lungs. This antioxidant quenches reactive oxygen directly and reduces cell death by 67 percent when applied immediately after a TBI event. When applied after three hours, glutathione reduced cell death 50 percent, which is still significant.

With the help of the recent research, we have the opportunity—and responsibility—to act quickly and immediately after injury with treatments that can save brain cells. Now that we know that brain injury isn't a single problem but a complex series of events and behaviors that varies among individuals—and that many of the single-mechanism drug treatments can be harmful or even deadly—we should take a different approach. We should look to nature's potent nontoxic nutrients and therapies to come back from a traumatic brain injury, because natural treatments are some of the most powerful and effective treatments for traumatic brain injury.

Why? Because the more similar the treatments are to natural processes, the less likely they are to cause further damage. By flooding the brain with nutrients that help correct dysfunctions of metabolism and circulation, we can start to repair the myriad kinds of damage caused by TBI. *By taking a more natural approach to the treatment of traumatic brain injury, we have the hope of better outcomes for those suffering terribly and can begin to turn the tide of this silent epidemic.*

If you or a family member suffer a traumatic brain injury, you need to know the steps to take to rescue your brain. In the following chapters, I will outline a step-by-step program similar to what is used at the Amen Clinics.

Because brain injury is a complicated process, the solution must encompass more than popping a pill. By you giving your brain and body what it needs, healing can occur for a serious injury that was once thought to be permanent. I will cover what nutritional supplements to take for acute as well as chronic brain injuries. I will describe what foods can heal brain injury and which brain exercises—from low-tech options like meditation to high-tech ones like brain games—are helpful in the healing process. I've found that certain hormones are a cornerstone of treatment along with solid sleep and vigorous exercise. I will also cover how to test for brain injury using imaging as well as lab testing.

Let me assure you that healing from brain injury is possible, which is why I will share stories of those who have recovered. My hope is that *Concussion Rescue* will be an invaluable resource that will help you or your loved one to make it all the way back, out of the fog and into the light of daily living—whole, complete, and your effective self.

Notes

1. Finch, Morgan TE. Systemic inflammation, infection, ApoE alleles, and Alzheimer disease: a position paper. *Curr Alzheimer Res.* 2007 Apr;4(2): 185–9.

2. Zhou, Xu, Zhang et al. Meta-analysis of APOE4 allele and outcome after traumatic brain injury. *J Neurotrauma.* 2008 Apr;25(4): 279–90.

3. Schwarzbold, Diaz, Martins et al. Psychiatric disorders and traumatic brain injury, *Neuropsychiatr Dis Treat.* 2008 Aug; 4(4): 797–816.

4. Koponen S, Taiminen T, Portin R et al. Axis I and II psychiatric disorders after traumatic brain injury: a 30-year follow-up study. *Am J Psychiatry.* 2002;159:1315–21.

5. Fann et al. Psychiatric illness following traumatic brain injury in an adult health maintenance organization population. *Arch Gen Psychiatry.* 2004 Jan;61(1):53–61.

6. Lu J, Marmarou A, Choi S et al. Mortality from traumatic brain injury. *Acta Neurochir.* 2005;Suppl(95):281–85.

2

THE BEST TREATMENT STARTS WITH AN ACCURATE ASSESSMENT

• •

BRIGHT MINDS Principles

When we assess for brain injury at the Amen Clinics we use our BRIGHT MINDS reminder:

Blood flow: Brain SPECT imaging can measure if the brain has sufficient or deficient blood flow, a critical element to know, especially if someone is presenting with symptoms such as chronic fatigue, depression, anger, or headaches.

Retirement/aging: As you age, the brain changes—and not for the better. It is sometimes difficult to know what is normal aging vs. what could be the start of dementia vs. what is impairment due to brain injury.

Head trauma: After conventional testing, such as a head CT scan, has ruled out a brain bleed, it is important to investigate further. We recommend taking a thorough history to learn of past brain injuries and also run a series of assessments using functional imaging, computerized evaluations, and brain games done with good old-fashioned pencil and paper.

Toxins: Functional imaging can show patterns consistent with the effects of toxins on the brain.

Mental health: Mental health problems should be thoroughly assessed, ideally through the use of functional markers and not just based on symptoms.

Immunity/Infection: We use laboratory testing and SPECT imaging to detect infections and inflammation that may be changing how the brain functions.

Only once we do a thorough evaluation and know what we are dealing with can we determine the best treatment plan and move toward healing.

• •

In a scene from the classic '80s film *Ferris Bueller's Day Off*, Ferris and his best friend, Cameron Frye, attempted to turn back the miles on the odometer of Mr. Frye's classic 1961 Ferrari 250 GT after a forbidden day of joyriding.

The boys placed the Italian sports car on blocks, shifted the gearbox into reverse, put a brick on the accelerator, and hoped that the odometer would spin backward, erasing all signs of their adventure. The engine revved up and the tires spun, but the car wasn't going anywhere. (And if you will recall, things did not end so well for Ferris and Cameron when the car slipped off its blocks and plummeted backward down an embankment.)

Do you ever feel like you're on blocks and your wheels are spinning—like you know something is not right, but you can't figure out what it is? Here's something you should consider if that's the case: even the most effective treatment won't work if it's targeting the wrong problem. When that happens and your health is suffering and you just can't get an accurate or complete diagnosis, the process can be frustrating and demoralizing.

Jane, a thirty-five-year-old patient of mine, had been diagnosed with "adult-onset ADHD," attention deficit/hyperactivity disorder, when she first came to see me. She had gone back to school to become a nurse and was struggling to keep up with her classwork. She felt overwhelmed, unorganized, forgetful, and depressed. She also complained of frequent headaches.

Her previous healthcare provider had prescribed Dexedrine, a stimulant, which helped a little, but not a lot, even at higher doses. Jane's life had become so unmanageable that her aging parents had to step in and support her.

In her patient history, Jane listed a number of concussions sustained as an adult in motor vehicle accidents, the most recent being a rollover accident. In the latter crash, Jane was able to walk away from the accident, although the emergency medical personnel that arrived on the scene insisted she go to the hospital for an evaluation. At the hospital, she was evaluated and released the same day.

Her SPECT (single photon emission computed tomography) brain scan showed evidence of a brain injury. When I met with her and her parents, her mother was shocked to hear the news.

"What brain injury? I don't remember Jane suffering from a brain injury," her mother said.

Jane had never suffered any symptoms typically associated with TBI after the accident, so there was no reason for anyone to suspect she sustained a brain injury.

Most people don't know that even mild brain injury can become chronic and cause long-term symptoms. The problem is this type of degenerative reaction is unpredictable. Statistics show, however, that 10 percent to 80 percent of those with a mild traumatic brain injury or concussion will continue to have chronic symptoms.[1]

Who recovers and who doesn't is based not only on what type of injury occurs, but also how it took place and the health of the person's brain at the time. This is a concept called brain reserve (or cognitive reserve), and refers to how resilient the brain is to damage. Basically, brain reserve is an indicator of whether you've treated your brain poorly or taken good care of your brain. Whether you have a good brain reserve or a poor one is a combination of factors, including genetics, whether you drink alcohol, eat a lot of trans fats, consume foods with high-fructose corn syrup, and get enough sleep.

For example, those who eat an unhealthy diet high in sugar and carbohydrates are probably more susceptible to the long-term effects of brain injury than someone eating a healthy diet filled with veggies and fruits. A rat study proved this point: for just four weeks, laboratory rats were fed a diet to mimic the standard American diet, which is high in sugar, carbohydrates, and fats. After being fed these foods, the rats had difficulty learning new information. This was tracked down to lower levels of BDNF—a gene known as brain-derived neurotrophic factor that provides instructions for the brain to make a protein that promotes the survival of nerve cells or neurons—in the memory centers of the rats' brains.[2]

Education is another protective factor for the brain. It's been shown that those with more education are less likely to show signs of Alzheimer's later in life.[3]

The good news is that brain reserve is not static; it can be improved at any stage of life. In a prominent Alzheimer's study conducted in Finland called the FINGERS study, researchers took 2,654 people ages sixty through seventy-seven who were at risk for cognitive decline. They improved their diet, put them on an exercise regimen, gave them brain-training exercises, and monitored their blood pressure, weight, and waist-to-hip ratio.

Guess what happened? The majority of the participants demonstrated a beneficial effect on cognition, specifically in the areas of memory, executive function, and psychomotor speed. Once again, taking good care of your body puts you on the path of taking care of your brain.

Brain Injury and Dementia

I understand that many of you reading this book have probably had some level of brain injury, and learning that a brain injury is one of the factors that make it more likely that you will have dementia later in life can be a frightening thought. Fortunately, you are not powerless. By strengthening your body and your brain, you will become more resilient mentally and less likely to suffer from dementia later in life. For those showing signs of developing dementia, I don't believe it's too late. Taking real, concrete steps toward healthy living now might move the onset of full-blown dementia back several years.

The suggestions in these pages will help you strengthen your brain and make you more resistant to any of life's blows—whether it is from another concussion or from dementia later in life. These strategies will also have a positive effect on cognition, taking you to the next level as far as your memory and focus are concerned, or helping to improve other brain-related symptoms.

Jane and her family were surprised that her present problems were the result of a long-ago injury, but they were heartened when I told them that now that we knew the problem, we could take the appropriate steps to fix it. If I had not evaluated her, Jane probably would have continued down the path of one medication trial after another. Figuratively speaking, she would have been spinning her wheels like Mr. Frye's Ferrari in *Ferris Bueller's Day Off.* What Jane needed was a comprehensive program to heal all parts of her brain, which is what will be discussed in later chapters.

The takeaway point in Jane's story is this: *Loss of consciousness is not a prerequisite for a traumatic brain injury.*

Diagnosing and Treating Mild TBI

A concussion is a form of mild TBI. According to the American Association of Neurological Surgeons, a concussion is defined as any change in mental status from a direct or indirect blow to the head, which may or may not result in external signs of damage. Symptoms may include "seeing stars" or feeling a little dazed after the impact.

I can't tell you how many patients come through our doors with classic concussion symptoms, having been told nothing is wrong by other healthcare providers—or that their symptoms are "all in your head." Well, they are all in the head—but sometimes those "imaginary" symptoms are due to a previously undiagnosed brain injury, even a mild one that occurred years earlier.

For example, when an ice hockey player rushes to the emergency room after a hit to the head, oftentimes imaging is performed, such as a CT scan of his brain. This is important to make sure nothing major, such as a brain bleed, is occurring. After the worst is ruled out, the injured person is typically told that everything is "normal" and rest is the primary treatment, and then they will recover. I'm not trying to put anyone down here, but what I think happens in this instance is more of a miscommunication than anything else.

In other words, when a doctor says that everything is "normal," what he or she means is the injury is not life-threatening, though you may have some damage that can't

21

be detected with the CT scan. The doctor is also saying that he or she hopes that your brain will heal and you will continue to survive through life with reasonably "normal functioning." In most cases of concussion, patients do recover with rest alone, and that's good.

What the patient typically hears, however, is very different: *What the doctor just said is that my brain and personality will return to the level of functioning exactly as it was before the accident.*

Sometimes functionality returns to normal, sometimes it doesn't. I'll admit my view may be skewed because I'm seeing all of those people that don't recover. When it doesn't, patients are left feeling shocked, along with their friends and family. And after that, they simply don't know what else to do but gamely face life "as is" with brain injury symptoms.

When mild brain injury symptoms persist, their attending physician often tells these patients three things:

1. There is nothing more that can be done.

2. Healing happens over time.

3. If healing does not occur over time, we can prescribe a stimulant to help with brain function, an antidepressant for mood swings, and muscle relaxers for sore muscles.

Sure, these patients can still function and get through life, but there are often anger, focus issues, balance problems, dizziness, tinnitus, depression, and fatigue. Sometimes an increase in anxiety or insomnia is a symptom.

In many cases, what is needed is a proactive, multifaceted plan to heal the brain, because I feel strongly that all three of the above suggestions are *false* more often than not. Here's why:

1. There *is* much that a person can do to heal from even a mild brain injury.

2. Time does not *necessarily* heal all wounds. While rest and high-quality sleep are important, sometimes rest alone is not enough to heal.

3. Sometimes stimulant medications are not the complete answer (though in some cases, combined with other healing approaches, they can help).

When you're told you're going to heal—and then don't—it can be crushing both emotionally and psychologically. When the symptoms continue, they are often attributed to other things. The brain-injured person starts to think things like, *Oh, it must just be stress,* or *I need more sleep,* or *I am just getting older.*

Because of a doctor's diagnosis, loved ones don't believe any of the subtle changes they are witnessing are tied to the original brain injury.

Let me clarify by saying that I am not trying to indict any doctor, especially emergency room doctors who are usually the medical practitioners treating brain-injured or concussed people who just had a fall or got a bump on the head. The main job of the ER physician is to keep a patient alive and rule out worst-case scenarios. These medical professionals also work in difficult, stressful environments.

That said, I do wish ER doctors would tell concussion victims something like this: "Though you don't have any brain bleeds or anything really serious, it is impossible to tell whether or not concussion-related symptoms will persist or even show up in a few weeks. For that reason, if you have any symptoms in the future, I want you to see your doctor."

My hope is that when the broader medical community learns more about the complexity of brain injuries, greater care will be taken immediately following a brain injury such as a bump to the head or a mild concussion. Instead of recommending just resting or avoiding stimulation, it would be helpful for patients to:

- Take a few simple supplements, such as fish oil (see more in chapter 5, First Aid for Your Brain)
- Exercise at appropriate levels and frequencies
- Follow some of the dietary suggestions in chapter 7, Can What You Eat Heal Your Brain?

These steps can make a big difference following a concussion, because there is far more to treating a concussion than just rest.

The good news is that most people *do* recover from a brain injury such as a concussion and feel better soon after the event. The problem is that a minority of people do *not* feel better, and months and even years following a brain injury they are asking why. They are depressed or have difficulty organizing, and the true cause of the problem is never discovered because they weren't assessed properly and were told they *didn't* have a brain injury.

If you or a loved one has symptoms after a brain injury, such as a change in personality or cognitive ability, don't be complacent: get help right away from a mindful physician who will take these symptoms seriously. Fatigue, depression, anxiety, menstrual changes, poor motivation, impulsiveness, migraines, and dizziness may be signs of a persistent brain injury that stubbornly does not want to heal.

If concussion is suspected, it's important to get a thorough evaluation. The routine concussion examination includes counting fingers, pupillary dilation, and response to light. These quick tests are done to rule out a brain bleed and whether or not a CT scan should be ordered. It's nearly impossible, however, to detect a very mild concussion by taking a history and a physical exam, which is why in chapter 5, "First Aid For Your Brain," I will discuss an approach for what to do if you should suspect a concussion, even after being evaluated by the appropriate medical professional.

Elements of a Good Brain Injury Assessment

So if it's so hard to assess whether there has been a mild TBI, what does an ideal brain injury assessment look like? Especially if the injury happened years ago? Here's a checklist I follow:

1. Start with a thorough history. Brain scans, lab work, and sophisticated cognitive testing are key tools in making an accurate diagnosis, but any good doctor knows that the most important piece of any good brain injury assessment starts with taking a thorough history of the patient. This means asking a lot of questions, and asking them over and over again—even if it seems repetitive.

One reason why it can be difficult to pinpoint a brain injury is that oftentimes, there is amnesia around the time of the injury. Also, as a society, we tend to minimize hits to the head and damage to the brain because we can't *see* the injury. A person on the street with a broken leg hobbling on crutches will typically get more sympathy than someone with a brain injury.

Nor are people aware that *a brain injury that happened weeks or even months ago could be the source of your memory or depression problems today.* (When a person comes to the Amen Clinics, our assessment goal is to ask them at least ten times if they have ever hit their head, either with or without a loss of consciousness. We need to know that information.)

When I first met Jeremy, he was a gregarious, likable, twenty-one-year-old jazz pianist who aspired to attend music school. He couldn't go to class, however, because of severe depressive symptoms and suicidal thoughts. He had been suffering with thoughts of taking his life since he was a sophomore in high school. He had also tried and failed to find relief from multiple antidepressant medications. But to his credit, he had also tried many therapies that can be effective, such as cognitive behavioral therapy, eye movement desensitization and reprocessing (EMDR), and hypnosis.

On his intake form, Jeremy had listed "none" under the head trauma section. When I looked at his brain scan, however, it was clear that there were asymmetrical findings of decreased activity in different areas of his brain. In particular, I had concerns about what I saw in the frontal and temporal lobes.

With his mother sitting next to Jeremy, I asked him if he was

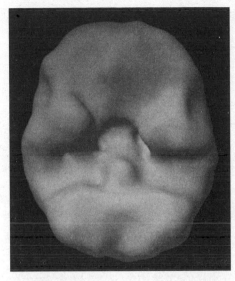

Healthy Brain

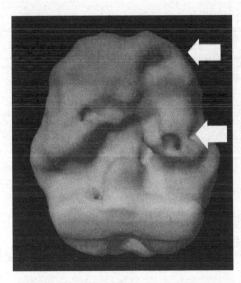

Jeremy's brain with arrows pointing to damage of the prefrontal cortex and temporal lobe.

sure he had never had a head injury. Remember, I knew that sometimes I had to ask that question, in a different way, ten different times.

"No," he said.

I asked him if he had ever fallen out of a tree, been bucked off a horse, crashed on a bike, dove into a shallow pool, been involved in a motor vehicle accident, or played contact sports. Each time, he responded that he hadn't done any of those things. But then he added something that caused my ears to perk up. "Well, I did play football from fifth to seventh grade," he admitted.

"Flag or tackle?" I asked.

"Tackle."

His mother piped in that he was quite small for his age and was often matched at practice against the coach's son, who was already a hulking form, standing nearly six feet tall. When I probed further, Jeremy described how he was regularly pulverized by the larger boy on the practice field and would often feel dazed when their training session was over. Then another revelation popped out: in sixth grade, Jeremy was diagnosed with ADHD and started taking Ritalin, a stimulant medication, and in seventh grade he had his first depressive episode.

Now we were getting somewhere.

Jeremy's second depressive episode happened when he was a sophomore in high school, and he'd had persistent problems ever since. After taking in this information, I told Jeremy and his mother that his brain injuries from playing football and getting hit like a tackling dummy had likely set him up to be highly susceptible to depression.

I put him on a program to help his brain heal, including an antidepressant based on his brain type. For the first time in many years, his suicidal thoughts began to lift. Two years later, Jeremy started attending a top music school. Just from looking at him I could tell that he was feeling optimistic, about his future.

Here's a key point: seeing Jeremy's brain injury on the SPECT brain imaging helped me ask better questions about what could be behind thoughts of killing himself.

2. Conduct cognitive testing. The second step after a thorough history is to start using additional testing methods, such as a cognitive test.

A cognitive test is any kind of examination that measures how your brain works. Your doctor might ask you to remember three words, and then ask you to recite them five minutes later. This type of test measures recall memory.

Psychologists have been using cognitive testing since the 1880s to measure different areas of mental functioning. A cognitive exam typically involves testing:

- Working memory
- Processing speed
- Attention
- Verbal memory
- Visuo-spatial recall
- Reaction time
- Executive function

Some of the seminal work by J. T. Barth and his group of researchers back in 1989 has become one of the primary ways to track cognitive symptoms in mild brain injury or concussions.[4] The tests may involve using a standard pencil and paper, or they may come from newer computerized testing. For example, the IMPACT (Immediate Post-Concussion Assessment and Cognitive Testing) measurement is an online test that, when interpreted by trained doctors, can help medical professionals decide when an athlete is ready to return to the field of play after a concussion. Under IMPACT, the athlete takes a baseline test before the season starts and then after each concussion.

WebNeuro is a more generalized Web-based test used to measure cognitive function. This test, which has been well-validated by the medical community for assessing many areas of brain function, takes about thirty to forty-five minutes and covers attention, processing speed, memory, mood, emotion identification, and self-regulation.

In fact, if you want to test your own cognitive function, you can do so by signing up to take WebNeuro on www. mybrainfitlife.com. The results are summarized and readable by the patient and clinician. This test can be repeated to assess ongoing progress and is one way to objectively measure how someone is recovering from a TBI event.

3. Undergo imaging. MRI (magnetic resonance imaging) or CT (computerized tomography) scans are normally used in brain injury assessment. At times, an MRI (or CT) scan will come back normal, even when a person has a brain injury. This is because MRIs and CTs look at structure, or the parts of the brain. Unless there is significant bleeding or a skull fracture, an MRI or CT will likely not pick up any damage. It's like taking a picture of a beautiful sports car that is pristine and perfect on the outside, but when you pop open the hood, the engine is a mess with parts either missing or broken. Therefore, this otherwise perfect-looking car either won't start or won't run at optimum performance. It can be the same with an injured brain.

Another type of scan is called SPECT (single photon emission computed tomography). The great thing about a SPECT scan is that it can look "under the hood" of your brain, rather than just at its structure. In other words, a SPECT scan looks at the activity of the brain and the brain's blood flow.

SPECT essentially describes three critical factors:

1. Which areas of a person's brain are working well

2. Which areas are working inordinately hard

3. Which areas are not working hard—or well enough

Below is a SPECT scan of a healthy brain. When we analyze a SPECT scan, we are looking for "holes," which imply decreased blood flow or damaged brain tissue.

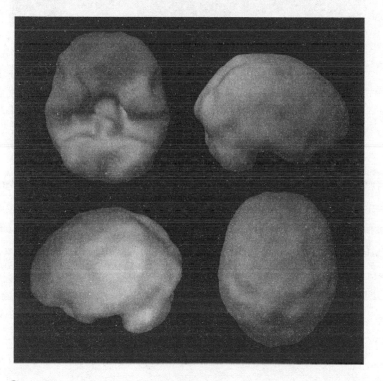

Compare this healthy brain scan with a scan of a retired NFL football player who spent sixteen years playing football and had concussive and sub-concussive hits resulting in chronic traumatic encephalopathy.

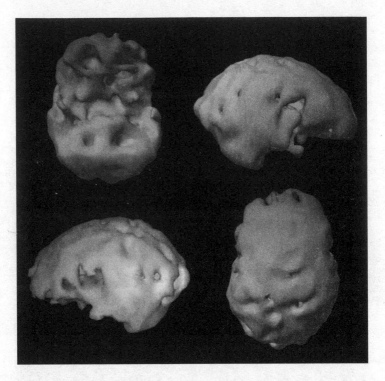

CT and MRI scans are critical to assess the worst damage after an acute brain injury when time is of the essence, especially when there is a brain bleed or a skull fracture. After the worst has been ruled out, however, these types of scans are nearly useless when compared to SPECT imaging. SPECT is able to do what an MRI (static) or CT simply cannot: measure brain function and the pattern of damage from even a mild TBI.

In a study conducted by Drs. Cyrus Raji and Rob Tarzwell, more than three hundred articles were reviewed to compare the efficacy of SPECT to MRI and CT for assessing brain injury. The study showed that if a patient is continuing to suffer from brain injury symptoms after three months or longer, SPECT imaging will pick it up 95 percent of the time. In addition, SPECT has a nearly 100 percent negative predictive value for assessing brain injury. This means that if a patient does not have a brain injury, SPECT imaging is helpful at ruling it out. This is especially important in diagnosing depression, fatigue, and memory problems due to psychological or biological factors, rather than from TBI. SPECT should be utilized when symptoms persist and an MRI or CT scan reveals "normal," but the patient doesn't feel totally recovered.

Not everyone can get a SPECT scan as the price tag can be prohibitive at around $4,000, and many types of insurance don't cover a brain SPECT scan for TBI, unfortunately. That is one of the reasons I am writing this book: I want to give you the tools to recognize TBI in other ways and point out that there are multiple ways to treat a brain injury.

In the next chapter, I'll take a look at some of the ways to assess for brain and body function after a TBI, including laboratory, cognitive tests, brain imaging, genetics, and the importance of a good history. These tests are key for helping to create an individualized healing plan for recovery from a TBI.

Notes

1. Brown AW, Elovic EP, Kothari S et al. Congenital and acquired brain injury. 1. Epidemiology, pathophysiology, prognostication, innovative treatments, and prevention. *Arch Phys Med Rehabil.* 2008;89(3 Suppl 1):S3–8.

2. Molteni R, Ying Z, Gomez-Pinilla F et al. A saturated-fat diet aggravates the outcome of traumatic brain injury on hippocampal plasticity and cognitive function by reducing brain-derived neurotrophic factor. *Neuro.* 2003;119(2):365–75.

3. Alexander GE, Furey ML, Grady CL et al. Association of premorbid intellectual function with cerebral metabolism in Alzheimer's disease: implications for the cognitive reserve hypothesis. *Am J Psy.* 1997;154(2):165–72.

4. Barth JT, Alves W, Ryan T et al. Mild head injury in sports: neuropsychological sequelae and recovery of function. In: Levin H, Eisenberg J, Benton A, eds. *Mild Head Injury.* New York, NY: Oxford University Press; 1989:257–75.

3

WHEN THE NUMBERS ADD UP

● ●

BRIGHT MINDS Principles

At the Amen Clinics, when we assess for brain injury and create a treatment plan, we refer to the BRIGHT MINDS mnemonic.

Inflammation: Inflammation can be measured in the blood and correlated with brain injury symptoms. We will employ measures described later in this book and then retest to measure inflammation down the line as symptoms resolve.

Genetics: Genetic testing can reveal susceptibilities such as the APOE4 allele which can tell you how suscep-tible you are to brain injury.

Head trauma: There is no perfect blood test for TBI, but there are tests that can assess for deficiencies and inflammation that can be treated.

Toxins: Toxins like heavy metals, toxic mold, and chemicals can be assessed as these can cause brain problems that slow healing.

Immunity/Infection: Testing for chronic infections like Lyme disease and Epstein-Barre Virus (EBV) can be helpful, as these may mimic many symptoms of post-concussion syndrome or TBI.

Neurohormonal deficiencies: Hormonal deficiencies are a key piece to address in order to recover from a brain injury. This topic is covered in the next chapter.

Diabesity: High blood glucose and prediabetes slow healing of the brain and worsen overall brain function.

Once we have a complete picture of the patient's health, we can determine the proper course of action.

• •

It was a brisk March day at Mont Tremont, a popular ski resort not far from Montreal, Quebec. Actress Natasha Richardson was enjoying a ski lesson on a bunny run called Nansen, known for its gentle slope and forgiving turns.

As sometimes happens while skiing on slick snow, Natasha took a tumble and hit her head. She seemed fine after she stood up and dusted herself off. She even walked around and chatted with others, although a member of the ski patrol recommended that she see a doctor right away. Despite the resort calling an ambulance to transport her to the hospital, she waved it off. "I'm fine," she said.

Early that evening, she called her husband, actor Liam

Neeson, who was on a film shoot in Toronto. "Oh, darling. I've taken a tumble in the snow," she said, as if the fall was just a trifle. Unfortunately, what seemed like an innocuous bump to the head proved to be much more than that. As it turned out, the blunt force trauma she sustained was quite serious. Natasha had suffered an epidural hematoma, which is an accumulation of blood between the skull and the brain. Her condition rapidly deteriorated. Tragically, she died two days later, leaving behind two teenage sons and a grieving husband.

How could a tragedy like this have been prevented? After all, Natasha had not shown any physical signs of a serious brain injury in the first few hours following her spill on the slopes. A CT scan or MRI would have picked up her brain bleed, but the hit to the head was so mild and there were no immediate symptoms. What's clear is that her death was a tragic reminder that science needs to come up with a simple test for TBI. Since there are hundreds of biomarkers released into the blood after a brain injury, you would think that a blood test is all that would be needed. However, the challenge is in figuring out which bio-markers are the most reliable and specific.[1]

I have good news to report: modern medicine is closer than ever to a quick, easy, and painless blood test that can detect acute TBI and categorize what type of damage has been done to the brain. In Europe, they are already using a simple finger prick that extracts enough blood to give medical providers a heads-up on whether the patient has been hit with a traumatic brain injury. For example, if you're in Germany during Oktoberfest, drink a few too many pints, and then trip and fall, hitting your head on the cobblestone street, medical personnel will prick your finger for blood to assess you for brain injury.

This blood test is called S100B, and although it has some shortcomings, the presence of blood tests like this one is a strong step in the right direction for assessing a TBI right after it happens.

Indisputably, the goal is to give paramedics, ER doctors and nurses, and even team doctors and trainers on the sidelines of athletic events a blood test that can be used when someone falls or takes a blow to the head. This is why I'm an advocate for developing this TBI blood test as soon as possible.

There's a Second Impact

Getting an accurate diagnosis of a TBI right away is absolutely critical, and sometimes every minute counts. One reason we need to assess right away, following any sort of brain trauma, is because of something known as "second impact syndrome." What is that?

When an acute brain injury occurs, the brain works overtime to rebalance itself at a time when it's very vulnerable. If a second brain injury happens, the results can be devastating, so those who believe they may have suffered a traumatic brain injury need to be vigilant and take it easy until they feel better, which is usually several days or even a week or more later.[2]

As important as it is to have a foolproof test for acute TBI, it is also important to test for the nutrients and hormones needed to heal. If the body lacks the proper nutrients or is dealing with residual hormonal problems, then healing from an acute injury is in serious jeopardy.

Fortunately, there are tests we can do to rule out nutrient deficiencies when it comes to assessing and evaluating treatment for a brain injury. Testing for and treating nutrient deficiencies can help not only brain injury patients, but also individuals suffering from a variety of brain-based problems such as depression, autism, ADD, and anxiety. A standard laboratory can assess for these deficiencies.

If you have hit your head, been told nothing is wrong and you're going to be fine, yet still have persistent symptoms that last more than several months, this would be a great time to have a panel done. What you want is an assessment of the amount of various nutrients within the body that are related to brain function. I normally recommend:

- **Lipid panel (cholesterol panel)**—which indicates cardiovascular risk factors. Total cholesterol for brain health should be above 150 mg/dL but not too much above 200 mg/dL.

- **Metabolic panel**—which measures liver and kidney function

- **Complete blood count (CBC)**—with special attention to:

- **WBC (white blood count)**—a low WBC is an indirect market of mineral deficiency or toxicity

- **MCV (mean cell volume)**—used to help assess nutrients. High normal levels may indicate B12 or folic acid deficiency; low MCV levels may indicate low iron

I also test for specific nutrients. If any of the nutrients listed are below the recommended amounts, then you may have found your susceptibilities to brain and body problems. I must state, however, that there is a difference between a true deficiency and a suboptimal level, which, if raised to an optimal level, may improve your chances of healing. The numbers listed have been obtained by clinical experience and from general medical consensus. Levels lower than the ranges indicated can cause neurological symptoms such as fatigue, anxiety, depression, difficulty with focus, and cognition problems. It's important to see your health provider so that you can discuss what the following nutrients are and what the numbers mean:

- **B12**—serum, should have levels above 600 pg/mL

- **zinc**—serum or plasma, should be greater than 100 ug/dL

- **copper**—serum, should be around the 100 ug/dL level

- **vitamin D** (both 25 OH and D3)—should measure between 60 and 80 ng/mL

- **ferritin**—should be at least 50 ng/mL

- **HSCRP**—an inflammatory marker, is optimal at <1 mg/L
- **homocysteine**—which is a cardiovascular risk factor and indirectly measures B vitamin status, should ideally be at the 6–8 umol/L level

Note: at least two days prior to doing any of these tests, stop taking a multivitamin and any supplements that contain zinc, B12, or copper. The reason is because these tests are measured as freely floating in the blood (serum), so if they are in your system, the test will measure the multivitamins and those supplements and not your body's correct measurements.

If you're wondering how these fundamental nutrients affect the brain, here is a brief overview:

Zinc

Zinc is important to brain health because this nutrient is a co-factor in more than two hundred biochemical processes in the body.

I have a special interest in zinc. When my youngest son, Cedric, was about nine months old, we realized he was more than just a colicky baby—he actually had severe developmental delays. He would become startled or frustrated and cry incessantly for up to forty-five minutes at a time. He hadn't started crawling and could barely sit up on his own.

My wife and I had him evaluated and learned, to our great sadness, that he met the State of Washington's criteria for in-home physical and occupational therapy. I decided to do what

I do for all my patients, which was check his zinc level, as well as several other key nutrients.

Bingo! That's when we learned that he was extremely low in zinc. We immediately started him on zinc supplements and noticed positive changes immediately. When the state evaluators came back the following week to give us their plan for future therapy, they almost didn't recognize him. They noted, for the first time, that he was beginning to move for them and was looking them in the eyes. Since then, he's still behind where he should be for his age, but he has made great and unexpected strides in his ability to process sensory information.

Zinc is helpful because it's also a co-factor in the production of dopamine, an element that helps with focus, concentration, mood stability, and impulse control. Zinc has been helpful in the treatment of ADHD as well as cases of depression that are otherwise treatment-resistant, according to several studies.[3]

We believe the increase of dopamine in Cedric's brain helped him become more active and aware.

One promising study showed that giving rats zinc after a traumatic brain injury improved their symptoms of depression behaviors. Cognitive improvements were also observed; the rats were able to complete water mazes at greater speeds.[4]

Cholesterol

Cholesterol is typically checked once a year as part of a routine physical. Most people know that high cholesterol counts can be a risk factor for heart disease. When conducting a brain assessment, however, you want to make sure that your cholesterol levels are not too low. Yes, *not too low*. Total cholesterol levels below 150 have been known to increase the risk of suicide and homicide in some TBI victims.[5] Also, when you look at the famous Framingham Heart Study, which began in 1948 and led to medical recommendations that lowering cholesterol reduces the risk of cardiac-related events, you can see that individuals with the highest cholesterol levels have higher cognitive functioning.[6] Of course, no one wants to sacrifice the brain for the heart, but there has to be a balance.

What is the connection between cholesterol and brain health? We know that the brain needs plenty of cholesterol, which is waxy and fatlike in appearance. This helps since the brain is 60 percent fat. Low cholesterol levels, I believe, make it difficult for some brains to recover from injury.

I must point out, however, that there is research from Johns Hopkins University showing that statin medications that lower cholesterol actually *improve* acute brain injury recovery by up to 75 percent. Researchers theorize that statins remove the excess cholesterol released from the brain after an injury to the head, kind of like mopping up. Since statins have other mechanisms of action, such as being anti-inflammatory, my guess is that those anti-inflammation properties are helpful for acute TBI.

However, I surmise that if we followed these patients throughout a long-term chronic recovery, we would find they would not do so well, because the brain needs cholesterol and fat for optimal functioning. Obviously more research is needed in this area.

I believe the optimal cholesterol level is between 160 and 180 mg/dL, unless you have other cardiovascular risk factors such as hypertension, diabetes, history of strokes, heart attacks, or obesity. That said, it's important to balance the healthful benefits of cholesterol for brain health with the cardiac risk for heart health and always work with your doctor, who will help you make these decisions. Trying to push cholesterol levels too low through the medical use of statins puts the brain at risk.

In the end, cholesterol is not the most important risk factor for heart disease anyway. A more significant risk factor for heart disease is inflammation, which is the signal that causes plaque to form. When in abundance, cholesterol will form these plaques more readily, so keeping inflammation levels low is important and can be achieved with the help of a good diet or supplements.

HSCRP

Highly sensitive C-reactive protein, or HSCRP, is a good way to measure inflammation throughout the body. The liver releases HSCRP if there are even small amounts of inflammation in the body. Inflammation may worsen the outcome of patients with TBI.[7]

If there is inflammation in the systemic circulation, this often correlates to inflammation in the brain and should be addressed. Keep in mind that HSCRP can also be elevated from an infection, a cold, or even from a rib out of place. If neither of these conditions exists, however, you could be suffering from inflammation in the blood vessels, which is harder to recover from.

Vitamin D

Vitamin D is a fat-soluble vitamin that's known as the "sunshine vitamin," but it's also a hormone the body requires to regulate the health of thirty different tissues and organs. Vitamin D activates and signals many different cells, including immune cells and neurons. The brain uses a lot of vitamin D every single day.

Research has shown a strong connection between vitamin D and TBI. In a study published in the journal *Clinical Endocrinology* out of Oxford University in England, 46 percent of patients with TBI were deficient in vitamin D, and those who were deficient had "impaired cognitive function and more severe depressive symptoms after a TBI."[8] That's why it's important for those who are at risk for a TBI to plan ahead and undergo tests to ensure that they have optimal vitamin D levels. For example, young athletes who play contact sports such as football, basketball, lacrosse, and soccer should all have their vitamin D levels checked and optimized prior to the start of their season.

I consider an optimal level of vitamin D to be between 60 and 80 ng/mL, even though the reference range is 30–100 ng/mL for most labs. Vitamin D is found naturally in very few foods. It is also produced when the ultraviolet rays of sunlight hit the skin and then miraculously trigger vitamin D synthesis. However, most people need to take a supplement.

Why? One possibility is that we have become photophobic,

meaning we avoid the sun due to the fear of skin cancer. We wear gobs of sunscreen when we go outside and make sure we stay indoors as much as possible. I think this approach is wise to avoid dreaded skin cancer, but it leaves us with having to supplement with vitamin D versus getting it naturally. As with most things, balance is the key.

Because many of us don't get enough sun, the recommended daily doses for vitamin D are higher than previously thought. For the majority of people, a dosage of 1,000–2,000 IU of vitamin D, maybe even 5,000 IU per day, can be recommended, unless you live in a hot, sunny location like the Mojave Desert.

However, as recently as 2005, some medical professionals feared that taking more than 800 IU of vitamin D could make the body toxic, causing elevated calcium levels that could lead to arrhythmias, kidney stones, and potentially death. Research since that time has shown that this is not true, and I can tell you that from testing thousands of my own patients' vitamin D levels, you can rest assured that higher doses are safe.

For most patients, I recommend as a minimum precaution taking at least 2,000 IU/day of vitamin D. This will provide a baseline level from which to build upon. However, we always check the patient's levels to see where they are at. If vitamin D levels are low, I then have them take higher-than-normal levels of vitamin D and then recheck to see if the levels are where they are supposed to be. It may take 10,000 IU/day for several months to fully optimize vitamin D levels.

Even at this level, toxicity is rare, but still, it can happen. Therefore, I don't recommend taking high levels of vitamin D for an extended period of time without being under the supervision of a doctor. According to the Vitamin D Council, 10,000 IU/day is the upper limit of safety.

If you're wondering if you can get all the vitamin D you need from getting more sunshine, the answer is yes, but it's complicated. Your skin tone, where you live on the planet, and how much skin is exposed are all variables when it comes to adding up your vitamin D production.

- According to the Vitamin D Council, an individual who is skin type III (someone who gradually tans) and exposes 25 percent of his body to the sun, at noon in Miami, for example, would probably need six minutes of exposure to the sun in the summer and sixteen minutes in the winter to make 1,000 IU of vitamin D. Keep those numbers in mind the next time you sunbathe.

- An individual with skin type V (someone who rarely burns and tans easily) would probably need around fifteen minutes of sun exposure in the summer and thirty minutes in the winter.

- In a northern climate like Boston during the summer, an individual with skin type III would probably need about one hour of exposure to the sun in the middle of the day to make 1,000 IU of vitamin D.[9]

- If you live above the 37th parallel (San Francisco, Denver, St. Louis, and Richmond, Virginia, for example), you need to know that during the winter months there's hardly any vitamin D–producing power from the sun because of the shallow angle of the sun's rays.[10]

Iron

Iron, best measured as ferritin in the blood, is important for neurological function. Although a person's ferritin level may be in the "normal range," the neurological system falters if the level drops below 50. Optimal levels are somewhere between 50 and 100.

One of the functions of iron is that the body uses it to make dopamine, a neurotransmitter—a chemical released by nerve cells to send signals to other nerve cells. Dopamine plays a role in controlling movement, which is why neurologists treating "restless legs syndrome" (RLS) will often give patients iron if their ferritin level is below 50; iron is needed by the body to make dopamine, and dopamine calms restless legs. According to Johns Hopkins researchers, "The single most consistent finding and the strongest environmental risk factor associated with RLS is iron insufficiency."[11] Dopamine also helps with focus and motivation. Low iron means less oxygen is carried to the brain, and when there is less oxygen, the body is lethargic.

Melissa, a patient of mine, was a fifteen-year-old girl struggling with concentration and focus issues. She had not responded well to initial treatments of stimulant medications, nor did she respond well to the supplements I'd given her. When her lab results came back, we found the reason why: her ferritin levels were at the bottom of the tank.

Melissa's low iron levels fit with her symptoms, including lack of motivation, which is a sign of a "sleepy" frontal lobe. When I directed her to take proper doses of iron, upward of 75 mg per day, her energy levels and ability to focus dramatically improved. I've seen similar results in hundreds of patients over the years.

It can take time for iron levels to normalize, and by time, I mean many months. Most people, with proper iron dosage, feel improvement within the first month or two. Many report significant improvement in three to six months.

Copper

Copper is another mineral necessary for brain function. Recent studies have found that the brain harbors the highest levels of copper in the body, along with high levels of iron and zinc. But having the proper copper level is crucial. Too much copper in the brain, however, may lead to various neurodegenerative diseases like Alzheimer's,[12] so too much of a good thing is not a good thing. Researchers at UC Berkeley discovered that *too little* copper is also a problem, because copper is needed for the development and firing of neural circuits in the brain.[13] It's a matter of balance and achieving the right level. Blood work gives an approximation of total body stores, so it's important to test and supplement as appropriate.

Homocysteine

Homocysteine, an amino acid produced by the body, is completely normal and necessary, but the presence of too much homocysteine is associated with heart attacks and strokes.[14] Homocysteine levels shouldn't be too low, either. The presence of this amino acid is the preliminary step to making cysteine, which is needed to make glutathione, an antioxidant capable of preventing damage caused by free radicals and heavy metals.

Treating the Whole Person

When it comes to patients with TBI, the goal is to treat the person—not her brain scan, or her lab value. I remind myself of that all the time, because I've learned over the years that the most individualized diagnosis and assessment produces the most efficient and effective improvements. The more I know about a person and can understand her, the better the treatment will be.

Many patients feel that by the end of their evaluation, I know more about them than anyone else, and in many ways, that's true. Spending time interviewing patients and reviewing their questionnaires and lab values helps me get a sense of the context and timeline in which to assess their brain functioning.

I'm grateful that I have SPECT imaging at my fingertips, which helps me understand how an individual's brain is functioning. One finding that I pick up often from SPECT imaging is not a pattern of brain injury but a pattern associated with toxins, infections, metabolic deficiencies such as anemia and hypothyroidism, and hypoxia or lack of oxygen.

The cause of toxicity may be obvious—it could be alcohol, cannabis, or other drugs. Other times, I have to dig deeper and order additional lab tests to figure out the cause of these problems. Sometimes the results point to something that many don't typically think of as causing toxicity to the brain, such as exposure to pesticides, solvents, toxic mold, or infections such as Lyme disease.

Many times, exposure to toxins is the cause of a person's problems. I often find, for example, that dentists, even if they don't use amalgam (mercury) fillings, end up taking them out of patients' mouths, which exposes them to these toxic metals. Removing amalgam fillings is an occupational hazard for dentists, which explains why many have accumulated toxins in their bodies. Hairdressers and manicurists have some of the highest on-the-job exposure rates to toxic chemicals. The application of these toxic chemicals, often in an enclosed space without proper ventilation, combined with hairspray, hair dyes, and other solvents and chemicals, is problematic. If you're in that line of work, make sure you get plenty of fresh air, take your breaks, and insist upon a well-ventilated work environment. If you have any symptoms often associated with toxicity, such as nausea, headaches, or dizziness, see your healthcare professional.

I also know how stress can be toxic to the brain. I was reminded of this when Rebecca, a forty-nine-year-old nutritionist, flew from rural Wyoming to our offices in Seattle for an evaluation. She was a highly intelligent, type A person with an extremely strong work ethic. She worked during almost all of her waking hours, seeing clients, researching, and working on her ranch, which lifted her spirits. A bonus was having a very healthy marriage.

At the time of her visit to see me, I noticed that she continued to see patients via Web-based videoconferencing—that's how dedicated she was. She told me that she worked endless hours, because she loved what she was doing and even fell asleep listening to lectures on her headphones at night.

About six months earlier, however, she had started experiencing excruciating headaches, which seemed to be getting more frequent and more intense. She was also walloped by fatigue so severe that she found herself dragging every day, no matter how much sleep she had gotten the night before. Most troubling to her, however, was that she was having difficulty concentrating and remembering what happened when she met with clients. During a seminar to advance her skills, her colleagues noticed she was asking them to repeat things.

Rebecca had seen an excellent medical doctor locally, who ordered a thorough blood workup on her and ruled out hypothyroidism, Lyme disease, autoimmune disease, cancer, hormonal problems, and menopause. A test for toxic mold came back negative.

As is often the case when the symptoms are unusual or unexplained, I was asked to have a look. Her diet was extremely healthy and she exercised regularly, but I noted that she was trying to do too much and often felt exhausted even after a short jog.

I wasn't sure what we were going to find when we conducted SPECT scans. When the results came back, I discovered that she actually had a healthy-looking brain, but there was evidence of a mild brain injury from a car accident twenty years earlier. She also had mild temporal lobe 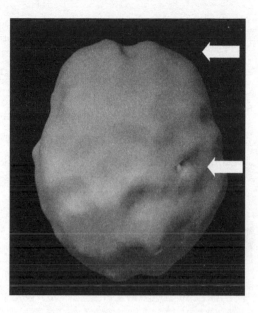 decreases in the medial section of her brain, where the hippocampus is located and is associated with memory.

This was evidence of an overactive brain. The results were not surprising, considering her passion about her work and her progress in her career. When I added the past injury to her brain from the car accident and her chronic stress, then it made sense that Rebecca had finally reached the point where she began exhibiting symptoms of ill-health. All she needed to do was to cut down her workaholic hours and get restful sleep as well as begin a treatment protocol for her past TBI.

Past brain injuries are like scars: in the present, they are areas of weakness. Rebecca certainly worked her brain very hard, and in the beginning she had enough innate brain function and resilience to overcome any deficits that the brain injury had caused, but as she aged and exposed her brain to chronic stress and overwork, she eventually hit the proverbial wall.

The effects of a brain injury can remain dormant until another assault on the brain—be it from injury, toxicity, or lifestyle. The injury is there, making the brain vulnerable; something triggers it and the symptoms appear. This was the situation in Rebecca's case. The good news, I told her, was that her brain was not toxic and she was not experiencing the early signs of Alzheimer's. Her sudden brain decline could be corrected, but all of her energy would have to be properly redirected toward rebalancing her body and mind and actively working to rest.

I knew that ordering her to relax and do less would give her her most difficult task yet. Writing her a prescription to take a vacation was easy on my part, but for someone who loves to work and owns her own business, it can be hard to slow down. I explained to her that actively doing things that decrease body and brain stress, however, would be the only way she could recover. "You're suffering from a classic case of burnout," I told her, "which is another way of saying that you're going through excess adrenal stress."

Stress can harm the brain in a very real way. The hippocampus, which is one of the memory centers, will actually shrink with excess cortisol (a stress hormone) production over a long period of time. This phenomenon has been widely discussed in scientific journals and textbooks,[15] and can actually be seen on an MRI. Rebecca's adrenal glands had been churning out cortisol for years. For any of us who thrive on this type of high-energy lifestyle, as robust and strong as our bodies are, they will eventually fail to adapt—which is what happened to Rebecca. She crossed the line of what her body could tolerate.

For Rebecca, pouring thousands of dollars into additional testing to look for obscure causes of complex neurological conditions would have been stressful and counterproductive. What she needed was to rest, eat a blood sugar–stabilizing diet, exercise lightly to moderately, get good-quality sleep, and take supplements that would help support her adrenal glands.

To her credit, she followed my prescription for turning around her health and was able to get her brain back in shape again and adopt a more stress-free way of life.

Unfortunately, Rebecca's story is not as common as I would hope. More often, I find signs of brain toxicity or infection and have to do a workup or refer the patient for further testing. This is because exposure to chemicals over time causes an insidious progression of neurological decline. While such a downward spiral isn't always correlated to pesticides, solvents, paints, or heavy metals, many times these toxic elements are the real culprits.

Genetic Testing

Genetic testing can help show what susceptibilities a person has, and how his or her body may be working—or not working well. For example, the APOE4 allele is known as the "Alzheimer's gene." Not only is a person more likely to be susceptible to Alzheimer's, but compared to someone who does not have this gene, they are more likely to suffer more severe effects from a brain injury.[16]

Imagine if all young athletes had the ability to know whether or not they had the Alzheimer's gene, which puts them at higher risk of having problems from a TBI. Would they want to play football? Would their parents allow them to even play football or some other head-banging sport like ice hockey? Knowledge is power, and at the very least you can be more cautious and proactive.

Other genetic tests include the MTHFR gene mutation test, which codes for an enzyme that processes folic acid. MTHFR is not an acronym for a curse word, but rather stands for methylenetetrahydrofolate reductase. In a nutshell, if you have this gene mutation, then it's highly likely that you have more difficulty processing folic acid (in supplement form) into the active form of folic acid called methylfolate.

You have one or two mutated copies of the MTHFR gene. Having this mutation also puts you at a higher risk for heart attacks and strokes. One reason may be because folic acid or methylfolate is needed to help lower homocysteine, and if homocysteine levels get too high, it irritates the lining of the blood vessels and contributes to clot formation, thereby increasing your chances of having strokes and heart attacks.

Taking folic acid (methylfolate), along with other B vitamins such as in a multivitamin, is usually sufficient to lower homocysteine levels. Just be sure that the folic acid is in the active form.

Further, without activated folic acid you are more likely to have depressive symptoms, attention problems, or increased cardiovascular risk. Green leafy vegetables such as kale, chard, and broccoli will supply you with the right forms of folic acid. But even if you eat these foods regularly, you may not be getting enough folic acid if you have the MTHFR gene mutation.

If you do end up having this gene mutation, know that it could represent the tip of the iceberg and that other gene mutations have interplay with this, including COMT (catechol-O-methyltransferase), CBS (cystathionine beta synthase), and MTRR (methionine synthase reductase). I know I'm being technical here, but genes related to methylation and natural detoxification processes in the body may be impaired and not working in harmony. Sometimes simply taking more folic acid (methylfolate) is helpful. But more often than not, because there are other genes or enzymes that may not be fully functional, a broader approach is needed.

Whatever you do, make sure you see a qualified doctor to help you figure out if there is more you can do to optimize methylation. The goal is to be proactive about potential treatments and to identify susceptibilities.

Finally, let me add that helpful resources that were created by a colleague of mine, Dr. Ben Lynch, are available at www.mthfr.net.

A Concluding Thought

If you're thinking that you should see a health professional for some of the issues I've described—lethargy, forgetfulness, loss of focus—know that the assessment is thorough and includes the following elements:

- History
- Cognitive testing
- Lab work
- Brain imaging
- Genetic testing

Work with your doctor or find one willing to work with you on some of the additional assessment pieces I've listed above. Armed with this knowledge, you can find the best treatment plan for you.

If you want to take a first step, then start with an online assessment through www.mybrainfitlife.com or by taking a memory test at www.memorylosstest.com/ free-short-term-memory-tests-online/?cst-report.

The brain is complicated, and adding some data points and figuring out what deficiencies you may have will not only give confirmation that there are problems, but also give you the beginning of a game plan to get your life and your brain back on track.

Notes

1. Mondello S, Muller U, Jeromin A et al. Blood-based diagnostics of traumatic brain injuries. *Expert Rev Mol Diagn.* 2011;1(1):65–78.

2. McCrory PR, Berkovic SF. Review second impact syndrome. *Neurol.* 1998;50(3):677–78

3. Piao M, Cong X, Lu Y. et al. The role of zinc in mood disorders. *Journal of Neuropsychiatry.* 2017 7(4), 378–86.

4.   Cope EC, Morris DR, Scrimgeour AG et al. Use of zinc as a treatment for traumatic brain injury in the rat: effects on cognitive and behavioral outcomes. *Neurorehabil Neural Repair.* 2012;26(7):907–13.

5.   Engelberg H. Low serum cholesterol and suicide. *Lance.* 1992;339(8795):727–29.

6.   Elias PK, Elias MF, D'Agostino RB et al. Serum cholesterol and cognitive performance in the Framingham Heart Study. *Psychosom Med.* 2005;67(1):24–30.

7.   Su S, Xu W, Li M et al. Elevated C-reactive protein levels may be a predictor of persistent unfavourable symptoms in patients with mild traumatic brain injury: a preliminary study. *Brain Behav Immun.* 2014;38:111–17.

8.   Jamall OA, Feeney C, Zaw-Linn J et al. Prevalance and correlates of vitamin D deficiency in adults after traumatic brain injury. *Clin Endocrinol (Oxf).* 2016;85(4):636–44.

9.   www.vitamindcouncil.org/about-vitamin-d/ how-do-i-get-the-vitamin-d-my-body-needs.

10. www.health.harvard.edu/staying-healthy/ time-for-more-vitamin-d.

11. www.hopkinsmedicine.org/neurology_neurosurgery/ centers_clinics/restless-legs-syndrome/what-is-rls/ causes.html.

12. Brewer GJ. Alzheimer's disease causation by copper toxicity and treatment with zinc. *Front Aging Neurosci.* 2014;6:92.

13. Dodani S, Firl A, Chan J et al. Copper is an endogenous modulator of neural circuit spontaneous activity. DOE/Lawrence Berkeley National Laboratory. *Proc Natl Acad Sci.* 2014;111(46)

14. Homocysteine studies collaboration. Homocysteine and risk of ischemic heart disease and stroke: a meta-analysis. *JAMA.* 2002;288(16):2015–22.

15. Bonne O, Vythilingam M, Inagaki M et al. Reduced posterior hippocampal volume in posttraumatic stress disorder. *J Clin Psy.* 2008;69(7):1087–91.

16. Friedman G, Froom P, Sazbon L et al. Apolipoprotein E-4 genotype predicts a poor outcome in survivors of traumatic brain injury. *Neurol.* 1999;52(2):244–48.

4

ASSESSING HORMONE IMBALANCE IN TRAUMATIC BRAIN INJURY

· ·

BRIGHT MINDS Principle

Neurohormone deficiencies: testing for and treating hormonal deficiencies is a cornerstone of TBI treatment.

· ·

"Hormones are the juice of life."

I will always remember Dr. Walter Crinnion, a well-known naturopathic doctor, saying these words at a conference that I attended. In many ways, it's true that hormones, when in balance, help you to perform your best, heal quickly, and feel vigor in life. When your body's hormones are in balance, the brain works optimally, and your energy is good. It's easier to relax and enjoy life to its fullest.

So here's an important point that I want to make right at the outset: *Some of the worst symptoms of brain injury can be traced back to hormone imbalances. In fact, they may be caused more by hormonal deficiencies than by actual brain injury itself. Fatigue, low libido, depression, insomnia, low motivation, anxiety, and poor concentration, as well a lack of recovery, may be related to the disruption of a functioning pituitary gland.*

The pituitary gland sits in the center of the brain, hanging from the hypothalamus by a slender stalk, and is called the "master gland" because it sends signals to most of the other glands in the body. The pituitary is susceptible to injury—just as other parts of the brain are—but perhaps more than other glands because of its odd shape. The pituitary gland looks like an upside-down ice cream cone, but its bulbous shape at the top makes it top-heavy. Whiplash or physical trauma can impact the blood supply to this fragile gland and cause considerable damage.

That's not a good thing, because the pituitary orchestrates the release of commonly known hormones such as estrogen, progesterone, testosterone, cortisol, and human growth hormone (HGH). This last one is key, because if human growth hormone levels are deficient, then it's going to be very difficult for the brain to "grow" or heal after a significant brain injury.

Statistics vary on how common hypopituitarism—which is defined as diminished hormone secretion by the pituitary gland, causing premature aging in adults and short stature in children—is after a TBI. The general consensus is that around a fourth of those with TBIs have hypopituitarism,[1] which is why I see this issue quite often in my practice. This is also why I believe problems thought to be due to brain damage may actually be a problem with the hormonal systems.

This concept is so important that I'm going to restate this one more time: *Many of the symptoms thought to be due to particular areas of the brain not working may actually be happening because of hormonal deficiencies.* I'm confident that fatigue, depression, and even anger may be due to low testosterone and not a brain injury. Anxiety, or in particular social anxiety, which means feeling overwhelmed in crowds or being put in situations with extra sensory stimulation, may be due to deficient pregnenolone, a chemical found in our bodies. Here's another example of a hormonal deficiency: if you're feeling light-headed when going from sitting to standing or having blood sugar problems, this may be caused by adrenal dysfunction.

When it comes to the pituitary gland, what's fascinating is that pituitary problems are dynamic, meaning sometimes they will get better and sometimes problems will arise in the months or even years following a TBI. This partly depends on the severity of the injury,[2,3] so checking and optimizing hormones is key to treating this problem. In particular, the primary deficits are human growth hormone in both sexes and testosterone in men and estrogen in women. For the rest of this chapter, I will be discussing natural ways to increase human growth hormone and testosterone and estrogen levels, but without the pituitary functioning properly, nothing's going to get better. That's why it's important to test and then correct all the hormonal deficits, which will give you a better chance for a damaged brain to heal.

Dr. Kevin Yuen, a neuroendocrinologist at the Swedish Neuroscience Institute in Seattle, was one of the pioneers in the field of pituitary research. Sadly, Dr. Yuen has since passed away, but the research he left behind informs us that approximately 30 percent of patients have some type of pituitary deficiency that can be seen in bloodwork two to three months after a TBI, in particular human growth hormone and testosterone deficiency.[4]

This finding is similar to the brain imaging study that Amen Clinics did on retired NFL football players demonstrating 100 percent damage across the surface of the brain.[5] (Another reason not to let your children play football.) You may not be aware that retired NFL football players generally have low testosterone levels. This may sound impossible since we all view these tremendous and larger-than-life athletes as mighty and strong, but once their playing days are over, upward of 30 percent of retired football players have low testosterone levels that lead to fatigue, depression, memory problems, and anger issues. They also have low human growth hormone levels, which results in low energy, depression, and cognitive difficulties. That's fairly normal for all men as they age, but that doesn't let women off the hook, because they need healthy levels of estrogen to preserve cognitive function, and their testosterone levels and estrogen levels drop at menopause.

When it comes to finding doctors who understand how to assess and treat hormonal deficits from a TBI, the name that comes to my mind is truly a leader in the field of endocrinology. I'm referring to Dr. Mark Gordon, a neuroendocrinologist who is the medical director at Millennium Health Centers in Encino, California. Dr. Gordon, a pioneer in testing and treating hormonal problems in brain injury patients, has worked with the military to treat countless veterans. He has also helped to start a foundation called the Warrior Angels Foundation to assess and treat veterans with TBI.

The driving force behind the Warrior Angels Foundation comes from a Green Beret patient he helped named Andrew Marr. Marr had been in Special Forces for ten years and suffered countless sub-concussive shockwave blasts to his head before he began showing signs of TBI. While serving in the military, he was on thirteen different medications, including meds for pain and depression, but they weren't helping. He struggled with alcoholism and depression, but it was the thoughts of killing himself that pushed him to reach out to Dr Gordon for help.

Andrew was tested and found to have severely deficient testosterone levels. When Dr. Gordon corrected those levels, it was like a veil had been lifted. Almost immediately, Andrew felt relief that he was *not* suicidal. He had his mojo back and a positive outlook again. Even more, he felt inspired to help other veterans who had suffered as he had. Andrew started the Warrior Angels Foundation with Dr. Gordon, and together they started raising money to treat veterans through this program. (Check out their website at www.waftbi.org/.)

Dr. Gordon has done an incredible job of bringing attention to the problem of hormone deficiency in brain injuries while training hundreds of doctors in how to assess and treat brain injuries using hormonal assessment and intervention. I say this with confidence, because *I* learned from Dr. Gordon, and his instruction completely changed the way I approach the treatment of wounded warriors and others suffering from brain injuries.

Now I'd like to shift gears and review the hormones that can become deficient following a TBI and what the implications are if these hormones remain low, as well as some strategies for how to correct them.

Before I go any further, however, I must issue a disclaimer that hormones are powerful and should always be used under a doctor's supervision, even over-the-counter hormones like DHEA, topical progesterone, and pregnenolone.

Testosterone

Testosterone is accurately assessed in a standard blood test, but what many forget is that there is an optimal range for testosterone based on age, with levels being higher during puberty and declining over one's life span.

Don't forget that women need some testosterone, just as men need some estrogen and progesterone, but not just as much.

The graphs on page 67 illustrate how testosterone levels decline with age for men and women.

A patient of mine, Trevor, was twenty-five years old when he was participating in a study-abroad program in Australia. He'd grown up always looking both ways before he crossed the street, but while Down Under, he forgot that drivers use the left lane. At a crosswalk, he looked left, saw no cars coming in his direction, and then took a step into the street. Unfortunately, he got hit by a car moving 50 kilometers per hour.

His head hit the windshield and the side mirror, and then his body hit the pavement like a Raggedy Ann doll.

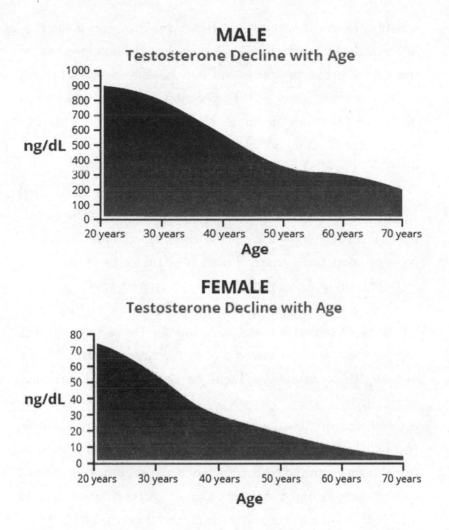

He immediately lost consciousness. Paramedics arrived and rushed him to the local hospital, where a broken leg was put into a cast and bandages were wrapped around his head, which had suffered scrapes and contusions. No testing was done for a traumatic brain injury, however.

Trevor returned to school but struggled with his

schoolwork and his memory. If he tried to read a page of homework, he had a terrible headache. He dropped out of the study-abroad program and flew back to Seattle, but his condition never improved. Depression, fatigue, and lowered libido were his "new normal." He was bummed that his life-long dream of going abroad to a university and traveling the world had been shattered.

I saw him two years after his accident because he'd tried twice to finish his coursework and graduate here in the States, but that wasn't happening due to depression and problems with concentration and memory. I noted that his leg had healed per-fectly, but his brain was still fractured in many ways.

One of the first things I did was to check his hormone levels. His testosterone was very low for his age, which was likely the cause of his lowered libido, depression, and fatigue as well. Testosterone is critical for optimal brain function, especially in males. There's a normal drop in testosterone around age fifty, which is termed "andropause" or "male menopause." This is the time when men typically start to have more cognitive difficulty such as forgetfulness or not feeling quite as sharp. Another sign of lowered testosterone is a lack of morning erections, which should normally happen because testosterone levels are highest in the morning and drop over the course of the day.

In younger males (those forty and under), testosterone from an external source—such as from injections or topi-cal application—is risky because it can suppress the testes' production of testosterone, which jeopardizes fertility. In

Trevor's case, I decided to treat him with something that would stimulate his body to produce testosterone.

I had several options for this, including a medication called clomiphene that stimulates the brain to produce testosterone. The beauty of this prescription medication is that it can be stopped at any time without issues, which reduces the risk of dependence. Even though clomiphene is derived from synthetic sources, it still works with the body by stimulating the production of testosterone.

For Trevor, his testosterone levels, which were at 300, zoomed up by 200 points to 500 points in two months. The positive effects were noticeable immediately: he had better focus, motivation, mood, and energy. I must state, however, that a level of 500 ng/dL is not optimal or enough for a healthy twenty-seven-year-old male.

Since he was feeling better, though, and wanted to make further changes, I got him to start implementing the exercise recommendations that I gave him. That, in addition to cutting the carbs in his diet, increased his testosterone by another 200 points. Now we were making some real headway, and Trevor felt better than he had even *before* his injury as far as mood, energy, and focus. Sure, I attribute many of these changes to his improved diet and exercise program, but I don't think he could have healed without the support of the critical hormone known as testosterone.

In summation:

- **Signs of low testosterone:** fatigue, problems with concentration, motivation, an increase in fat-to-muscle ratio, memory difficulty, and anger.

- **Options for treatment:** testosterone injections, testosterone cream, testosterone stimulators— herbal options such as *tribulus terrestris* and ginseng, hCG (human chorionic gonadotropin) injections, clomiphene, interval training, and a low-carb diet.

Progesterone

Perhaps one of the greatest stories regarding brain injury–related research and possible natural treatments is the story of progesterone.

Progesterone may be one of the most effective treatments for TBI, yet it's hidden in plain sight. Why progesterone? I begin by saying that progesterone is typically thought of as a female hormone, and with good reason. Researchers have found female rats—and especially those at the highest peak of progesterone in their menstrual cycles—survived TBIs better than male rats.[6]

The question flummoxing researchers is this: Why does progesterone help in brain injury? We know, from research, that progesterone levels are highest when a woman is pregnant and her fetus is bathed in high levels of progesterone, which protects the developing unborn child and grows tissue. I can't imagine anything better for acute brain injury than protection and growth.

Over three hundred preclinical trials on progesterone and brain injury support its use as a treatment, but we are still lacking effective human trials. Typically, a preclinical trial is a study done on animals, while clinical trials are done on humans. So far there have been three clinical trials done on around a hundred human subjects. Each of them shows improvement for TBI.

For instance, one of the first larger scale studies in humans was called the "ProTECT" Study done in Georgia at a Level One trauma center and demonstrated a decrease in the death rate by 50 percent in those subjects given progesterone within eight hours of injury.[7] Even more exciting is the prospect of combining progesterone with vitamin D, another potent nutrient for the brain. Several studies, including a clinical study out of Iran, showed that this combination reduced the risk of death from 30 percent to 13 percent in TBI subjects.[8]

These were smaller human trials, so the next step is to repeat the treatment with a larger patient population. Unfortunately, two large-scale studies of progesterone for one thousand TBI patients resulted in them showing no improvement. My thinking on why these studies failed to demonstrate efficacy is because more than just one hormone is needed to facilitate the healing of a TBI. Unfortunately they left out a key ingredient: vitamin D. A total package is the best route to helping TBI patients, a package that includes feeding the brain that has low energy with a ketogenic diet; providing vitamin D for a deficient brain and body; and providing antioxidants to support the healing process.

From what I've seen, progesterone in these studies for acute TBI was used more like a medication because of its anti-inflammatory and neuroprotective properties with patients who would otherwise die or be in a vegetative state. This is very different from testing an individual for hormonal and nutrient deficiencies and then replenishing their nutrients, which works very well for chronic TBI. These are two entirely different applications because one is for acute cases and the other is for chronic cases.

The take-home point is this: the doses of progesterone necessary for TBI patients are similar to those that a woman receives in the late stages of her pregnancy. This level of treatment is more useful for acute versus chronic TBI, but could be helpful for chronic TBI, especially if there is chronic inflammation and more so in women.

The combination of progesterone with vitamin D in the study mentioned above is significant because it goes back to the idea that the multiple-mechanism problem of brain injury requires a multi–mechanism of action treatment, which vitamin D does beautifully. Progesterone and vitamin D complement each other well and work to manage inflammation without completely eliminating it, because some level of inflammation is needed for tissue repair and healing. These hormones also help with reduction of glutamate, which is the excitatory neurotransmitter that causes further damage when released after injury. Further, together these nutrients help with the management of calcium. Calcium is a useful mineral, but can be too much of a good thing, because improper use causes more damage to the brain. Like glutamate, some calcium is helpful for nerve conduction, but too much can trigger cell death, which is a devastating consequence.[9]

For these reasons, I do not prescribe progesterone for more than eight weeks after an acute TBI in either men or women, because there doesn't appear to be any long-term benefit.

After that time frame has passed, I switch patients over to other therapies based on their specific deficiencies so as to not overdo one specific hormone that may disrupt the entire system. I *would* continue long-term therapy for men or women if there was some secondary benefit, such as for anxiety or insomnia. For example, progesterone is typically calming and relaxing, but just for brain injury treatment after initially using progesterone acutely for the first six to eight weeks.

In cases of mild TBI, progesterone could be equally effective, but I'm not aware of any specific trials on mild TBI and progesterone. I realize that the mechanism of injury is thought to be largely the same without as much inflammation, cerebral swelling, and widespread damage to tissues.

Women have just as many or more hormonal impairment problems after a TBI or concussion, including menstrual irregularity. Sometimes, their monthly period stops altogether after a brain injury due to pituitary problems. Furthermore, there can even be difficulty getting pregnant or maintaining a pregnancy after a brain injury.[10] One study showed that 48 percent of women lost their period for up to sixty months post-TBI while 68 percent had abnormal menses.[11] They tend to have a profound lack of estrogen/progesterone and testosterone as well as growth hormone. Women, of course, also have the same post-TBI problems as men, including a lack of focus, depression, and low energy.

In summation:

- **Signs and symptoms of low progesterone:** anxiety, insomnia, fibrocystic breasts, bone loss, infertility, premenstrual syndrome, and irregular menses.

- **Options for treatment:** the consumption of herbs that increase progesterone levels, such as *Vitex agnus-castus* or chaste tree berry. Medication options include oral progesterone sublingual drops or capsules and topical cream.

Human Growth Hormone

Human growth hormone (HGH) is one of the most important hormones to check for after a brain injury. If growth hormone levels are low compared to a person's age, this can be the reason why he or she is not recovering.

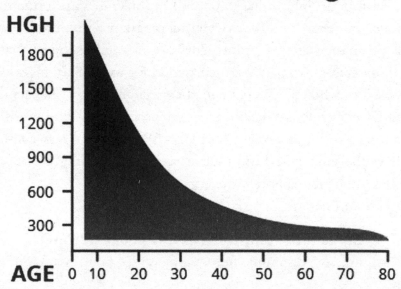

74

Human growth hormone is highest when you're young and then drops gradually over time. A drastic drop in human growth hormone due to head injury is going to slow the rate of healing dramatically.

Human growth hormone promotes the healing of tissues of all types, including brain cells. HGH, if low, leads to depression, fatigue, and difficulty concentrating, along with a general lack of energy and vigor for life. Working with an endocrinologist or doctor knowledgeable in hormone assessment and therapy can help, and a good first step is checking human growth hormone levels.

HGH is most accurately measured by testing an indirect marker called IGF-1 and IGFBP-3, because this measures a more average level, whereas human growth hormone itself is released in small bursts throughout the day and is harder to detect accurately through a simple blood test. If IGF-1 is low or in the low normal range, the next best step is to see an endocrinologist who can perform a more involved and accurate test of HGH known as the glucagon stimulation test.

The release of human growth hormone in the body is highest in puberty and declines as a person ages, but it must be stated that a spike of growth hormone can be stimulated at any age by intense exercise and a lower-calorie diet. In fact, interval training, which I discuss more in chapter 11, Exercise and Traumatic Brain Injury, increases human growth hormone by at least 450 percent of normal levels for up to two hours, which is like having a growth hormone injection.[12] If there is at least partial pituitary function, intense exercise may be enough to stimulate growth hormone release. This may be why those individuals who do intensive exercise often look younger and more vibrant.

The research on supplements for increasing human growth hormone is scant.[13] I do think it is reasonable, however, to consider adding in several specific amino acids before a workout and at bedtime to support growth hormone release. To do this, find a product that contains the amino acids L-arginine, L-ornithine, and L-lysine, often called tri-amino. The usual dose of four capsules containing approximately 1,200 mg of L-arginine and 1,200 mg of L-ornithine and 900 mg of L-lysine, taken at bedtime and before intense exercise, gives you the greatest chance at increasing levels.

My endocrinology professor, Dr. Dirk Powell at Bastyr University, once told me about a fourteen-year-old boy he had seen who had low levels of human growth hormone and short stature. Dr. Powell prescribed him tri-amino, but the patient did not follow up for several years. When Dr. Powell saw him next, he was seventeen years old and unrecognizable in that he had grown to over six feet tall. It's certainly possible that he simply was a late bloomer and had his growth spurt later, but he surpassed both of his parents in height.

A word of caution: oral dosing of specific amino acids to increase human growth hormone is highly variable in response. I have found this to be the case clinically as well as in situations where retesting levels of human growth hormone will sometimes be sufficient from taking amino acids and performing interval training, but at the same time may require further interventions.

If you're considering taking hormonal support for a TBI, find a doctor who has been trained by Dr. Gordon to help assess and treat you.

In summation:

- **Signs and symptoms of low human growth hormone:** increased body fat to muscle ratio, fatigue, depression, and a lack of vitality.

- **Options for increasing human growth hormone:** doing interval training and taking tri-amino. You can also consider taking formulas that increase human growth hormone like secretropin and sermorelin or taking actual human growth hormone injections.

Adrenal Gland Function

The adrenal glands are small glands that sit atop the kidneys. Part of what the adrenals do is to help you to manage stress and emotionally taxing events through the use of cortisol. Cortisol is a stress hormone that is normally released in a diurnal pattern over the course of the day to maintain basic body processes such as keeping blood sugar stable between meals. Cortisol is released from the adrenal glands, which are stimulated to do so by a release of the hormone adrenocorticotropic (ACTH) from the pituitary gland. Cortisol is released in short bursts approximately six to ten times over the course of the day, with levels being the highest in the early morning and at noon.

Under periods of stress, however, this number doubles and there are many more bursts. Examples of stressors are pain, hypoglycemia (low blood sugar), depression, anxiety, infections, sleep deprivation, and fear.

The adrenal glands can help the body handle these acute stressors, but when the stressors become chronic and unrelenting, the adrenals can compensate for only so long before their initially robust response to these stressors begins to lessen and it becomes very difficult to handle any stressor. What I see time and time again in my office are people who are true type A personalities who boast that they can work a forty-to-fifty-hour workweek while going to school and raising a family all at the same time. One day, however, they found that they were not able to do it all anymore and they "hit a wall," "crashed," "had a nervous breakdown," and could not continue to handle the relentless burden of stress piled on themselves every day. These individuals had, over time, stressed their bodies and brains to the point where eventually they could not hold up the weight of stress that was beating down on them. Since people must rest periodically, rest can only be delayed for so many months or years before the body starts to break down. Everyone has a breaking point, which happens when the body forces them to rest.

I recall a patient who told me that she wished she would get some kind of serious disease or injury so that she would be forced to take time off of work.

"Why?" I asked. "Can't you simply take a vacation like a normal human? Or request time off?"

She didn't have an answer for me, and that's because it's

hard to stop and slow down, especially if you're "addicted" to moving fast and staying busy. There have been times when I've literally written on my prescription pad: "Vacation two weeks, no substitution permitted," which would then give them permission to take the time off they needed.

I will talk more about how you can restore normal adrenal and cortisol functioning momentarily, but the short answer is that it all comes down to personal boundaries and self-care. Saying "no" to more work and "yes" to more relaxation, family time, and exercise is what fills up the well of energy and restores adrenal function.

It's not uncommon for cortisol levels to be elevated immediately following a brain injury. As I stated, cortisol is considered a "stress" hormone, which is why the adrenal glands work overtime to release more cortisol following a TBI event. Studies have found that 30 percent of patients are agitated after a brain injury, and when these patients were tested, 70 percent or more had excess cortisol levels in their blood.[14,15] However, if the pituitary gland is damaged, there can be significantly reduced levels of adrenal hormones because the pituitary stops stimulating the adrenal glands to release cortisol. In studies assessing for adrenal insufficiency soon after a TBI, rates of adrenal insufficiency range between 23 percent and 50 percent.[16]

Signs of adrenal stress or decreased adrenal function are fatigue, lack of motivation, a paucity of initiation, an intolerance to hot or cold, easy fatigability, difficulty concentrating, and symptoms of hypoglycemia (low blood sugar) and hypotension (low blood pressure).

Sometimes this pattern is reversed and cortisol levels are released throughout the entire day due to stress. If cortisol levels remain high at night, it can be very tough to sleep because the body is "amped up."

Adrenal gland function can be tested in several ways, including through a four-point cortisol test that measures the level of cortisol over the course of the day. Cortisol can also be measured by an early morning blood draw and sometimes an afternoon blood draw. It can also be measured with a twenty-four-hour urine measurement. For ease with patients, I will typically do a serum cortisol test in the morning.

The person who has had the brain injury is not the only one who suffers adrenal stress. Caregivers and family members can be expected to go through emotional and physical changes as well, and would benefit from the recommendations in this chapter.

There are several ways to help adrenal gland function. The first is to reduce stressors. This may sound simple, but keep in mind that there are many hidden stressors in life, including both physical as well as emotional stress.

Keep blood sugar levels stable by eating protein, healthy fats, and low-glycemic carbohydrates (vegetables) at each meal and snack during the day. You especially want to keep your blood sugar from dropping because that will cause a surge of cortisol and adrenaline. Getting at least seven and a half hours of sleep a night is also critical. As I've mentioned earlier, sleep is when your body produces human growth hormone and other hormones that your brain needs in order to repair and heal. Your adrenal glands simply don't have much chance of recovering if you're sleeping six hours a night or less and skipping meals.

In addition to these foundational elements, adaptogenic herbs are an important key to improving adrenal levels as well as cognitive functioning. Adaptogenic herbs are plants that help us "adapt" to stress of any type. For example, panax ginseng helps increase mental as well as physical endurance. I have many patients who take ginseng and stop having severe hypoglycemic episodes when it gets close to mealtimes and feel they have significantly improved focus. One patient of mine noted that the "fog lifted" after starting a combination of these herbs.

Ashwaganda is a great adaptogenic herb, especially if there is an element of anxiety. In Sanskrit, the words *ashva* and *gandha* refer to smell, and I must say, this root herb does have kind of a horse sweat smell to it, but I prefer to think that this herb gives you the strength of a horse.

I believe healing adrenal gland function is possible. My specific recommendations are:

- Getting seven and one half hours of quality sleep each night
- Maintaining stable blood sugar by consuming protein, low-glycemic carbohydrates (vegetables), and healthy fats at each meal
- Decreasing external stressors, meaning being around people who build you up versus those who bring you down
- Setting boundaries, both internally and externally

- Saying "no" to tasks that drain energy
- Saying "yes" to things, people, and opportunities that build you up
- Exercising to "blow off" excess cortisol each day
- Perhaps trying one or two of these adaptogenic herbs
    a. Ashwaganda extract, 250 mg/capsules, 1–2 capsules twice daily
    b. Panax ginseng extract, 500 mg/capsules, 1–2 capsules in the morning
    c. Siberian ginseng extract, 500 mg/capsules, 1–3 capsules in the morning
    d. Rhodiola rosea extract, 250 mg/capsules, 2–3 capsules in the morning

Here's one more idea to help you minimize your stress response. It's called "Challenging the ANT."

The term *ANT* was brilliantly coined by Dr. Daniel Amen and stands for automatic negative thoughts. We all have them, those thoughts that predict the worst, and cause us to be consumed by worry and self-doubt. Having these negative thoughts puts us in a state of stress and can trigger the release of cortisol. Challenging the ANT involves identifying automatic negative thoughts and challenging their truth, and once you do that, the power of the thoughts are lessened. This cognitive behavioral therapy technique is strongly effective at turning down the volume on that negative voice inside your head.

Thyroid

The thyroid is the gland of metabolism and energy. This is why patients who complain of always feeling fatigued flock to their doctors to ask for their thyroid to be tested with the hope that a messed-up thyroid is the cause of their weight gain, feeling tired and sluggish, or feeling cold.

More times than not, however, the thyroid-stimulating hormone (TSH) test comes back "normal" or "within the reference range." When that happens, as it often does, the patient's dreams and hopes that relief would be as simple as taking thyroid medication are shattered.

However, a full thyroid panel is critical to assess true thyroid function, and often the "normal" values aren't optimal, especially if there are thyroid symptoms. One of the thyroid tests that isn't done often is called reverse T3. Under certain conditions, like chronic stress, the body will produce high amounts of reverse T3, which makes the metabolism slow down, the body temperature drop, and the brain turn off. This physical state is ideal for a hibernating bear but not for a human being trying to live in today's fast-paced world. Because the brain is so metabolically active, turning down the metabolism even a little bit can have a huge impact on brain function.

In summation:

- **Symptoms of thyroid problems:** fatigue, feeling cold, depression, slowed mental capacity, and edema (swelling).

- **Options for treatment:** conducting screening tests to assess pituitary and hormonal function after brain injury such as:

  LH/FSH

  Cortisol

  Testosterone, free and total

  Estradiol

  Estrone

  Progesterone

  IGF-1

  IGFBP-3

  DHEA-S

  Pregnenolone

  Free T3

  TSH

  Free T4

  Reverse T3

  Prolactin

  AM cortisol

  PSA (prostate specific antigen for men)

Hormone optimization is an integral component in the treatment of TBI. Checking for low hormones is the first step, and then finding the right doctor to correct and treat those low levels is the second. Restoring hormone levels to their optimal pre-injury and youthful levels results in remarkable results in treatment.

Notes

1. Schneider HJ, Kreitschmann-Andermahr I, Ghigo E et al. Hypothalamopituitary dysfunction following traumatic brain injury and aneurysmal subarachnoid hemorrhage. *JAMA*. 2007;298(12):1429–38.

2. Tanriverdi F, Ulutabanca H, Unluhizarci K et al. Three years prospective investigation of anterior pituitary function after traumatic brain injury: a pilot study. *Clin Endocrinol (Oxf)*. 2008;68(4):573–79.

3. Tanriverdi F, De Bellis A, Ulutabanca H et al. A five year prospective investigation of anterior pituitary function after traumatic brain injury: is hypopituitarism long-term after head trauma associated with autoimmunity? *J Neurotrauma*. 2013;30(16):1426–33.

4. Kelly DF, Chaloner C, Evans D et al. Prevalence of pituitary hormone dysfunction, metabolic syndrome, and impaired quality of life in retired professional football players: a prospective study. *J Neurotrauma*. 2014;31(13):1161–71. doi: 10.1089/neu.2013.3212. Epub 2014 May 8.

5. Raji CA. Abnormally low blood flow indicates damage to NFL players' brains. *J Alz Dis*. 2016;53(1).

6. Stein DG. Progesterone exerts neuroprotective effects after brain injury. *Brain Res Rev*. 2008;57(2):386–97.

7. Wright DW, Kellermann AL, Hertzberg VS et al. ProTECT: a randomized clinical trial of progesterone for acute traumatic brain injury. *Ann Emerg Med.* 2007;49(4):391–402.

8. Aminmansour B, Nikbakht H, Ghorbani A et al. Comparison of the administration of progesterone versus progesterone and vitamin D in improvement of outcomes in patients with traumatic brain injury: a randomized clinical trial with placebo group. *Adv Biomed Res.* 2012;1:58.

9. Bano D, Nicotera P. a2+ signals and neuronal death in brain ischemia. *Stroke.* 2007;38(2):674–76.

10. Ripley DL, Harrison-Felix C, Sendroy-Terrill M et al. The impact of female reproductive function on outcomes after traumatic brain injury. *Arch Phys Med Rehabil.* 2008;89(6):1090–96. doi: 10.1016/j.apmr.2007.10.038.

11. Colantonio A, Mar W, Escobar M et al. Women's health outcomes after traumatic brain injury. *J Womens Health (Larchmt).* 2010;19(6):1109–16. doi: 10.1089/jwh.2009.1740.

12. Stokes KA, Nevill ME, Hall GM et al. The time course of the human growth hormone response to a 6 s and a 30 s cycle ergometer sprint. *J Sports Sci.* 2002;20(6):487–94.

13. Bucci L, Hickson JF Jr, Pivarnik JM et al. Ornithine ingestion and growth hormone release in bodybuilders. *Nutr Res.* 1990;10:239.

14. Jackson RD, Mysiw WJ. Abnormal cortisol dynamics after traumatic brain injury. Lack of utility in predicting agitation or therapeutic response to tricyclic antidepressants. *Am J Phys Med Rehabil.* 1989;68(1):18–23.

15. Cohan P, Wang C, McArthur DL et al. Acute secondary adrenal insufficiency after traumatic brain injury: a prospective study. *Crit Care Med.* 2005;33(10):2358–66.

16. Llompart-Pou JA, Raurich JM, Pérez-Bárcena et al. Acute hypothalamic-pituitary-adrenal response in traumatic brain injury with and without extracerebral trauma. *Neurocrit Care.* 2008;9(2):230–36.

5

FIRST AID
FOR YOUR BRAIN

●●●●●●●●●●●●●●●●●●●●●●●●●●●●●●●●●●

BRIGHT MINDS Principles

Blood flow: After a hit to the head, blood vessels can be damaged, leading to decreased blood flow. This must be addressed as a core piece of healing from brain injuries.

Inflammation: Inflammation is related to chronic symptoms of brain injury. The nutrients used in a brain injury protocol must address inflammation in multiple ways. Particularly helpful nutrients are omega-3s (EPA/DHA), curcumin, vitamin D and vitamin C.

Head trauma: Using targeted nutrients at the right doses is a key to healing from concussions or brain injuries, and the faster you act, the more brain cells are saved.

●●●●●●●●●●●●●●●●●●●●●●●●●●●●●●●●●●

At seventeen, Thomas played each lacrosse game like it was his last.

Balls to the wall was his motto. Thomas not only loved the fast pace, snap passing, and the teamwork that were the hallmarks of lacrosse, but he also fed on the attention and prestige that the fastest-growing sport in high school competition gave him.

During his senior year, Thomas was expected to carry the team since he was the best player on the field. Early in the season, however, he sprung up to fight for a pass and got tangled with another player. He lost his balance and couldn't find his feet as gravity took over. Thomas hit the ground awkwardly with the back of his head. Even though he was wearing a helmet and slammed into a relatively softer synthetic turf, he still saw stars.

Play stopped. Thomas remained immobilized as his trainer ran out to have a look. After he was helped to his feet, Thomas's vision became blurry. Loud ringing filled his ears, and his head pounded like a jackhammer.

Thomas was escorted off the field and took a seat on the bench. The ringing in his ears and the pounding in his head were not good signs. The trainer held up three fingers on his right hand.

"How many fingers am I showing?" he asked.

"Three."

The trainer studied him further. "I think you're done for the day," he said. "Better safe than sorry."

Concussions are difficult to diagnose, so the trainer was playing it safe. He knew that if Thomas had any mental changes after hitting his head, then his brain had been damaged to some degree. Since the trainer was aware that this was Thomas's fifth concussion in four years, the young player had to be held out. There was no other option.

For Thomas, having another concussion and being told that he couldn't play were the worst pieces of news possible. He had several college scholarship offers on the table, but if he was concussion-prone and not allowed to play anymore, those offers would be rescinded and free schooling would be out the window. There was a lot riding on whether he played, from the financial implications to the health risks of yet another concussion. Was it worth it?

Thomas thought back to his first concussion. The headaches and sensitivity to light lessened considerably after one week. However, with each successive concussion, Thomas noticed that his headaches and sensitivity to light took longer to dissipate. By the time he suffered his *fourth* concussion, his symptoms didn't improve for a good month.

His latest concussion was more of the same. He took a few days off from practice, but the reality was that he had to get back on the lacrosse field if he wanted that college scholarship. The trouble is that Thomas knew he was far from 100 percent. He wasn't as sharp in the classroom and forgot things. Good study habits kept his grades up, but everything was a huge mental effort—from his class work to remembering his role when his lacrosse team was on offense.

But still, he played.

Let's rewind the end of this scene again, but this is the way I wished things would have played out.

. . . he sprung up to fight for a pass and got tangled with another player. He lost his balance and couldn't find his feet as gravity took over. Thomas hit the ground awkwardly with the back of his head. Even though he was wearing a helmet . . . he still saw stars . . . loud ringing filled his ears, and his head pounded like a jackhammer.

Thomas immediately recognizes the signs of concussion as he's assisted off the field. When he sits on the bench, instead of his trainer asking him how many fingers he's holding up, the trainer opens a first aid kid that contains capsules of an amino acid derivative and antioxidant known as N-acetyl cysteine (NAC), vitamin C, and the herbal extract curcumin. He grabs the correct number of capsules and hands them to Thomas along with a water bottle, motioning for him to take them.

Then the trainer reaches into his kit for glutathione cream to apply to the youngster's temples and neck. After rubbing the cream onto the skin, the trainer shines an LED light device on the back of Thomas's neck for several minutes to stimulate a healing response and decrease inflammation. The light signals the cells to stop the cascade of events that produce inflammation that leads to brain injury and instead begin to repair nerve cells.[1]

The trainer isn't done yet. He then reaches for his smartphone and finds a concussion app—yes, there is one—known as the Concussion Recognition & Response (CRR), which has a list of questions that the trainer can ask that can reveal whether someone has had a concussion. This app can also keep a record of previous concussions.

Here's what I see happening after the game. When Thomas gets home, his father mixes him a special high-fat shake that will help his body produce ketones, which are substances that the body makes when fats are broken down for energy. At the same time, his mother prepares a plate of mixed green vegetables (kale, spinach, and broccoli) topped with a superior protein source like lightly broiled Alaskan salmon, and finally garnished with a whole avocado and a handful of olives.

For the next few days, Thomas will continue to eat a diet very low in carbohydrates, high in vegetables, high in healthy oils such as avocado and olive, rich with protein from wild salmon also high in omega-3 oils and moderate in protein. This type of diet shifts his body into a state of nutritional ketosis, which means the body's cells don't have enough carbohydrates to burn for energy so they turn to burning fat instead. (I'll discuss this way of eating in chapter 6.)

The next time Thomas sees his family doctor, which should happen within a week of the concussive event, an evaluation includes the examination of all his cranial nerves and his balance system. He passes those tests with flying colors, prompting his doctor to encourage him to stay hydrated, rest, take Advil or aspirin for headaches, and call if his symptoms worsen. Back at school, Thomas visits with the team trainer, who does additional balance testing on him to further assess for concussion.

At this point, let's assume Thomas shows some deficits from his concussive event. He continues taking the supplements and waits to exercise for forty-eight hours, and then starts with some standard aerobics. His symptoms (headaches) return when he's on a treadmill, so he reduces intensity and shortens his workout for the day.

After a few days, his mind is clear and sharp again and his energy has returned to normal. He resumes his regular routine of exercise and schoolwork. He takes his maintenance and concussion preventive supplements each day. He makes sure to eat a healthy diet low in processed foods and high in healthy fats, proteins, and vegetables, with small amounts of more complex carbohydrates like steel-cut oatmeal and whole grain pasta and starchy vegetables like sweet potatoes and corn.

After this concussion, Thomas had only a slight headache for a couple of days. After a couple more days of rest, he was ready to play lacrosse again and catch up on his schoolwork with no further symptoms.

Of course, anyone can see the desirable difference in the outcome of scenario 2. Even taking one or two of the steps I outlined would be an improvement over the current standard of care for concussions.

There are many research-based methods for treating acute moderate to severe traumatic brain injuries. Most come from studies performed on animals and some on humans, so they may not be unequivocally translatable to mild traumatic brain injuries in humans. In my view, however, these treatments do not cause harm and may help.

Some people may think what Thomas and those around him did in scenario 2 seems like overkill; they would argue that he may have recovered without taking the steps I described. But I would counter that it only seems like overkill because the protocol he followed was so different from what is currently being done—and because we cannot actually see the internal brain injury that has taken place.

It's hard to believe, but strapping on a seat belt once seemed like overkill to people. Now it's the norm—not to mention the law. Decades of use, as well as research, have confirmed that the simple act of using a seat belt saves countless lives. When it comes to concussions, trainers, coaches, parents, and military leaders may think that it's too much preparation or effort to administer extended initial treatments after every perceived concussion, but think about how the brain is our most important asset. Why would we *not* take simple measures to avert extensive damage just because we can't *see* the injury? I hope this point produces a paradigm shift toward the prevention of the long-term problems of brain injury in our society.

The medical profession has made wonderful strides in improving our lives, as well as saving us from severe traumatic brain injury, but clearly more help is needed. Currently, there are few recommendations to actively reduce long-term damage and begin the healing process. Each year, a million athletes hear the same mantra from their health professional: "Rest, avoid stimulation, and hope for healing and recovery."

But we can do better.

We must do better.

I don't want to minimize the work of many healthcare providers. In the United States, we have some of the smartest and most progressive neurosurgeons in the world. Due to their dedication, lives are saved every single day, and the death rate from brain injury has dropped from 40–50 percent to between 20–30 percent.[2]

At the same time, though, treatment methods are not progressing and improving as fast as they should, even as we continue to make advances to save lives. For instance, we know that approximately four times as many people who suffer from mild TBI don't report their symptoms as compared to those who do, which means they never receive treatment.

We need to educate the public about the importance of seeking out appropriate care, even though many physicians counsel their patients to rest and take it easy until symptoms ease. But over the years, I've seen many, many patients whose concussion symptoms continue for years. They've seen medical professionals, but their physicians didn't know how to help them get better.

This is why I see a huge need for a book like *Concussion Rescue*. There are treatment options that my team and I have developed at the Amen Clinics that I believe can make a real difference in the lives of thousands of people who've suffered a traumatic brain injury.

This information needs to get out. Yes, what I talk about will be controversial in some quarters, because any treatment or new way of looking at things attracts criticism—until these treatments are shown to work and become accepted as standard of practice. More research is needed, but that will come.

I have seen thousands of patients who are still suffering many of the same symptoms they reported at the time of their initial brain injury—headaches, depression, concentration problems, fatigue, irritability, dizziness, vision problems, and tinnitus. Their conditions have not improved with time. Even if they score within "normal" criteria after testing, it may not be normal for *them*, so they continue to have symptoms that are difficult to test for, such as fatigue, headaches, and dizziness.[3]

Research varies, but around 50 percent of patients report symptoms for up to three months after a mild traumatic brain injury such as a concussion, and 10 percent to 15 percent report symptoms for as long as one year.[4]

So consider this question: What if we, like Thomas's trainer, could immediately do something that increases the rate of recovery from traumatic brain injury, similar to how we routinely treat a sprained ankle with rest, ice, compression, and elevation?

There are many things that anyone, not just physicians, can do to help immediately after a traumatic brain injury. For instance, Theodore Roth, the young researcher at Stanford, discovered that when applying glutathione to an injured mouse's skull, the result was decreased cell death by 67 percent when applied immediately after the injury and by 50 percent when applied after three hours. Roth's findings tell us that we have a window of time in which to act and apply the effective principles of treatment to the damaged brain.

That said, I can imagine the day when I'm in the grandstands, watching a football or soccer game, and I see a player take an especially hard hit to the head. After being tended to, he's taken to the sidelines and given a mix of the potent antioxidant N-acetyl cysteine (NAC) and vitamin C (very important for brain protection and repair) that will ameliorate some of the cell death and inflammation that has already started but hasn't been felt or seen yet. This simple step can help avoid a future of debilitating fatigue, depression, anger, and higher risk of dementia.

What is the typical protocol for treating a concussion today? Depending on the severity of the injury, a physician may or may not order the injured party to get an MRI or CT scan. For sure, the doctor will direct his patient to go home, get rest, withdraw from all physical activity and possibly school or work for one week, take Tylenol for headaches, and stay hydrated.

If the injury is severe enough to require surgery, then the patient will often have to stay in the hospital for rehabilitation to relearn walking, talking, and other activities of daily life. The Stanford Concussion and Brain Performance Center, ahead of the curve in many respects, recommends aerobic exercise as soon as possible to accelerate recovery and encourages people to look for support such as through peer groups.

These recommendations, however, assume that the brain has all it needs to recover and that nothing is getting in the way of that recovery. I would not leave it up to chance if one of my loved ones suffered a brain injury. I would do everything I could to ensure that his most precious asset—the brain, which is the focal point of who he is—has all of the necessary nutrients it needs to fully recover its daily functioning. Not addressing the source of damage is like adding more sandbags instead of closing the floodgates.

Quenching Inflammation

In chapter 1, I described how there are many different physiological processes happening all at once after a traumatic injury to the brain. They are:

1. Inflammation at the neuronal level, which is damaging to neurons

2. A reduction in cellular energy and abnormal electrical signaling

3. Cells that are rapidly dying

In addition to recommending rest and avoiding excess stimulation, I would like to see doctors direct patients to take targeted nutrients to quench inflammation and recommend diet strategies that will help heal the brain rather than worsen inflammation.

Keep in mind that a nutrient or therapy for treating brain injury must fulfill the following criteria:

- The nutrient or therapy must have broad mechanisms of action and work on multiple targets.

- The substance or therapy must be nontoxic even in high doses.

- Each substance or therapy must be designed to fulfill a different purpose, but many of the mechanisms of action are overlapping and synergistic.

I would like to see the application of brain science immediately to every athlete, motorist, pedestrian, and cyclist as well as every man, woman, and child suspected of having a brain injury. I do this for my own family. My children are a bit small to go on family bike rides, but I carry a "TBI first aid kit" with me on hikes or stash it in the car just in case any of us would—God forbid—find ourselves in a situation where I would need to apply immediate intervention.

Of course, I would use my TBI first aid kit in a Good Samaritan situation as well, such as if I came upon someone who fell off a bike or slipped on the ice. I would use my kit to help that person since the passage of time equals the number of brains cells lost. My goal isn't to replace 911 or emergency medical care, but to do minimum preventative care while waiting for trained EMTs to arrive.

I recommend that you have a TBI first aid kit on hand. I'm providing a handy chart below to help you know what to include in the kit. And if you're wondering if it's a hassle carrying such a kit on a hike or bike ride, then let me put you at ease. You are not taking the entire kit with you, and besides, stashing a bit of extra gear in a backpack is a minor bother compared to the good you can do.

My TBI first aid kit is designed to be portable and do the most good in the shortest amount of time. Here is what you should include in your kit, along with a basic information about timing and dosage. You should copy this list and keep it in your kit at all times so that you don't have to have to recall all the information from memory during an emergency. *And remember, this first aid kit does not in any way take the place of emergency medical care.*

I recommend that the TBI first aid kit includes all the

nutrients that should be taken immediately in a small ziplock bag or an empty vitamin bottle. In a separate ziplock bag, measure out 1 tablespoon of the MCT oil powder or 6 caps and 1 tablespoon of flavored branched-chain amino acid (BCAA) powder. Some companies make the premixed medium-chain triglycerides (MCT) oil/ketones in convenient packets as well. Then you should have a "home kit" where you have enough supplements to follow the TBI first aid kit protocol for at least one week.

The TBI First Aid Kit

Emergency Travel Kit
to Be Taken Immediately

8 NAC (500 mg/cap)—Dosage should be 50 mg for every kilogram of body weight—this dosage is based on a 175-lb person
2 curcumin (500 mg/cap)
2 vitamin C (1,000 mg/cap)
2 vitamin D (5,000 mg/cap)
1 tablespoon MCT oil powder or 6 caps
1 tablespoon flavored BCAA powder

Take everything immediately after injury, ideally within one to three hours, but no later than twenty-four hours after injury. MCT and BCAA powder should be mixed into eight to ten ounces of water. The kit relies on the injured party's ability to swallow pills, which can be problematic for young children, but even kids can take the MCT powder and BCAA. The idea is to use these ingredients in addition to getting a thorough checkup to make sure that nothing serious like a brain bleed or skull fracture has occurred. Remember, loss of consciousness is not required to have a serious injury to the brain.

First Aid Kit for At-Home Use

The following nutrients are recommended for the week following injury. The amounts indicated are enough to last one week.

50 **NAC (500 mg/cap)**
19 **curcumin (500 mg/cap)**
14 **vitamin C (1,000 mg/cap)**
16 **vitamin D (5,000 mg/cap)**
14 **Omega-3 fatty acids (EPA>DHA
    800 mg/cap)**
MCT oil powder
Flavored BCAA powder

DOSAGE

Days 1–4

Twice a day take:

4 **NAC**
2 **curcumin**
1 **vitamin C**
1 **vitamin D (5,000 mg/cap)**

1   **Omega-3 fatty acids (EPA>DHA 800 mg/cap)**

3   **tbsp MCT oil powder**

Three times a day take:

1 **tbsp BCAA powder**

Days 5–7

Twice a day take:

3 **NAC**

1 **curcumin**

1 **vitamin C**

1 **vitamin D (5,000 mg/cap)**

1 **Omega-3 fatty acids (EPA>DHA 800 mg/cap)**

3 **tbsp MCT oil powder**

Three times a day take:

1 **tbsp BCAA powder**

Another consideration in acute TBI scenarios is the use of progesterone, which we learned about in chapter 4, "Assessing Hormone Imbalance in Traumatic Brain Injury." Work with a doctor on this one and consider using 2–4 mg/kg daily for the first month after an acute injury.

As a foundation, a potent multivitamin is crucial for TBI recovery because the brain will be needing *all* the vitamins and minerals it can get. For example, having sufficient magnesium in the bloodstream is important to balance the damaging influx of calcium that happens after a brain injury. A multivitamin that contains at least 50 mg or even 100 mg of a highly absorbable magnesium such as magnesium glycinate or citrate is ideal. Methylfolate and Methyl B12 will be necessary to make new DNA to then build proteins and neuronal cells.

I know this has been a lot of information, but having your own TBI first aid kit at home is a great idea, especially if you have active kids who can slip and fall on their heads or get injured in a headbutting sport. I'll describe these brain-supporting nutrients in greater detail in the next chapter.

Having a TBI plan on hand, one that is based on a logical application of science to the problem of concussion or a TBI, will give you a tool to help navigate the complex puzzle of knowing what to do and how to help.

Employing these nutrients and the ones I describe in the next chapter are almost like strapping on a seat belt before going out onto those freeways. It's a way of increasing the likelihood of recovery if the head is rattled or injured.

Always take care to avoid any risk of head injury, because prevention is the best way to ensure that a long-term injury won't happen to you or a loved one. These nutrients are one strategy to increase healing time, but it may not be enough, especially if the spine is moved out of alignment or the hormonal system is damaged. Further workup will be needed as well as an ongoing strategy.

I'm aware that many of you reading this book are not

dealing with acute problems but have TBI symptoms that have been present for months or years, and you're looking for help. In the next chapter, I'll describe additional approaches for chronic TBI.

Notes

1. Naeser MA, Saltmarche A, Krengel MH et al. Improved cognitive function after transcranial, light-emitting diode treatments in chronic, traumatic brain injury: two case reports. *Photomed Laser Surg.* 2011;29(5):351–58.

2. Lu J, Marmarou A, Choi S et al. Mortality from traumatic brain injury. *Acta Neurochir.* 2005;95(Suppl):281–85.

3. Levin HS, Gary HE, Eisenberg HM et al. Neurobehavioral outcome 1 year after severe head injury: experience of the traumatic coma data bank. *J Neurosurg.* 1990;73(5):699–709. See also McAllister TW. Neurobiological consequences of traumatic brain injury. *Dialogues Clin Neurosci.* 2011;13(3):287–300.

4. Spinos P, Sakellaropoulos G, Georgiopoulos M et al. Postconcussion syndrome after mild traumatic brain injury in Western Greece. 2010;69(4):789–94. doi: 10.1097/TA.0b013e3181edea67.

6

NATURAL TREATMENTS FOR CHRONIC TRAUMATIC BRAIN INJURY

• •

BRIGHT MINDS Principles

Blood flow: After a hit to the head, blood vessels can be damaged, leading to decreased blood flow. This must be addressed as a core piece of healing from brain injuries. Botanical medicine such as ginkgo help to increase blood flow to the brain.

Inflammation: Inflammation is related to chronic symptoms of brain injury. The nutrients used in a brain injury protocol must address inflammation in multiple ways. Omega-3s (EPA/DHA), curcumin, vitamin D, and vitamins C and E are helpful.

Head trauma: Using targeting nutrients at the right doses is a key to healing from concussions or brain injuries.

• •

By now, I'm hoping that you understand the importance of a TBI first aid kit and having all of the nutrients accessible so they can be taken as soon as possible after a traumatic brain injury like a concussion.

But I also understand that most of you reaching for this book are well past the acute phase of brain injury. What you need help with now is healing from a brain injury that you've been struggling with for months or, more often, years. You may have been told there's nothing else that can be done, so you just have to live with your symptoms.

No! There is hope, and I say this with confidence, because I've seen thousands of patients who have had chronic symptoms of brain injury over the years recover and resume life as before.

Although the bulk of the research literature focuses on nutrients and treatments for acute TBI, some of the mechanisms of injury in chronic TBI are similar to acute TBI, so it makes sense then that many of the nutrients used for acute TBI will help those with chronic TBI even though there hasn't been a lot of long-term research and trials done on them.

I look forward to the day when we will have data on chronic TBI and what works best with treating the condition. In the meantime, while patients continue to have loss of function and suffer with extreme fatigue and behavioral issues, I'm going to do whatever is in my power to help individuals with the best information we have at this time. The research may be scant, and there are still gaps in what we know, but I'm reminded of the saying, "Don't let perfect get in the way of the good." My feelings can be summed up in this manner: if I can help you get an improvement in function with something that has a nearly zero risk, why not consider it?

Each of the following vital elements can mitigate the devastating effects of a traumatic brain injury. I'll start with the items in the TBI first aid kit and introduce some key nutrients that you may or may not have heard about before:

N-Acetyl Cysteine (NAC)

Here's a semi-complicated medical study explanation, but stick with me on this one, because it's important.

In 2013, NAC was used in a study aiming to ameliorate the effects of brain injury on soldiers who suffered head injuries while in combat. This double-blind, placebo-controlled trial took eighty-one military personnel and enrolled half to receive NAC; the other half received the placebo. Both groups were assessed and treated within twenty-four hours of artillery-blast injuries that had resulted in a mild traumatic brain injury. Their symptoms included headaches, confusion, memory loss, and insomnia.

Those slated to receive NAC were given a loading dose of 4 grams, and then 2 grams twice daily for four days, and then 1.5 grams twice daily for three days. After the one-week trial, 86 percent of the NAC group experienced a complete resolution of their symptoms, whereas only 42 percent of the placebo group had resolution of their symptoms.[1]

NAC is extremely helpful in TBI, because it's a broad-acting antioxidant. Over fifty human trials have shown its effectiveness for a variety of conditions.[2] This nutrient helps to produce glutathione, which is a potent antioxidant produced by the body from three amino acids: cysteine, glutamic acid, and glycine. The topical applications of glutathione, which were used in the mouse study cited previously, clearly reduce cell death after acute TBI in animals. Studies haven't yet confirmed if topical application of glutathione reaches the human brain, however.

NAC has many functions in the body, including acting as an antioxidant and an anti-inflammatory. Another widely effective use of the glutathione-producing properties of NAC is how it helps the liver filter harmful substances. In fact, NAC is such a powerful liver detoxifier that it has saved the lives of many individuals in the emergency room who've overdosed on Tylenol, an over-the-counter medication that can be deadly when taken in quantities over the recommended dose.

Curcumin

Curcumin is an extract of the Indian spice turmeric, which is the ingredient in curry that makes it bright yellow. Plants have hundreds of chemicals with many gentle mechanisms of action; the main one that curcumin is used for is quenching inflammation and swelling. In a study of brain injury on mice, curcumin reduced interleukin-1, an inflammatory chemical released in the brain, as well as aquaporin-4, a water channel that, when activated, lets the floodgates open and causes swelling in the brain.[3]

In addition to the high-quality professional or

pharmaceutical-grade brands like Pure Encapsulations and Vital Nutrients, there are also over-the-counter brands of curcumin such as Jarrow, Life Extension, Doctor's Best, and Natural Factors.

I like curcumin when it's formulated with black pepper because of the way absorption is enhanced. When formulated with a fatty substance called phytosome, curcumin gets into the brain faster.

MCT Oil Powder

Medium-chain triglycerides, in a powder form, are commonly derived from coconut oil, palm oil, and dairy fats. They spur the production of ketone bodies.

Be aware that some of the MCT oil powders on the market have trace amounts of dairy protein (casein or sodium caseinate), so if you have a dairy sensitivity, you will want to go with one that does not contain dairy. MCT oil powder tends to have less gastrointestinal troubles and diarrhea associated with it than MCT oil liquid. But either of these can cause GI upset, especially on an empty stomach.

Branched-Chain Amino Acids

Neurotransmitter imbalances are a common problem after a traumatic incident to the brain, and branched-chain amino acids are well suited to balance this deficiency.

Branched-chain amino acids are used most often by athletes to speed recovery and encourage muscle growth. I have used BCAAs after longer runs or intense workouts and they do help, but they taste terrible. I choked down the unflavored kind (blech!) until I was able to find the flavored option, but look for ones that contain no artificial flavoring or coloring. Powder form is the best way to get the higher doses necessary for effective TBI treatment. I recommend mixing the powder in water or including the substance when making a "brain shake," which I will describe how to do shortly.

After an injury, in addition to helping restore the balance of neurotransmitters, branched-chain amino acids also speed recovery and healing of brain cells. In a study examining both mild and severe TBI, the researchers saw a reduction in branched-chain amino acid levels in test subjects' bloodstreams.[4] It was shown that by replenishing branched-chain amino acids, there was a restoration of more normal neurotransmitters as well as helping in energy metabolism and repair.[5] However, while I do recommend including BCAAs in your TBI First Aid Kit, do have some caution about taking them daily for an extended amount of time, as taking too much of one combination of amino acid may suppress and block the absorption of another, such as tryptophan (the precursor to serotonin), leading to a depressed mood.[6]

Vitamin D

Vitamin D, as I described earlier, is more of a hormone than a vitamin and is essential to brain health, and specifically to helping alleviate the symptoms of traumatic brain injury. Vitamin D interacts with over one thousand genes and neurons in the body and the brain.[7] Vitamin D has an immunomodulating effect, meaning it calms excess immune reactions such as inflammation and improves deficiencies in the immune system.

Vitamin D promotes calcium influx, or absorption, which is critical for bone health. But this hormone also regulates calcium absorption, and this is very important in the context of TBI, because calcium dysregulation (meaning too much calcium) leads to cell death, thought to be one of the major causes of secondary brain injury. Vitamin D's ability to balance calcium levels and provide neuroprotection may be why, and how, this vital nutrient helps prevent the damage that is part of the inflammatory cascade.[8]

But can there be too much of a good thing when it comes to vitamin D? An interesting study in the medical journal *Hormones and Behavior* demonstrated that low and moderate doses of vitamin D had more neuroprotective effects than higher doses. In fact, researchers found that the higher doses either didn't help or were less effective. Personally, I think it's reasonable to give a dose of vitamin D of 10,000 IU per day as soon as possible after injury.[9]

Also keep in mind that the overall strategy with vitamin D is to check your level and then optimize it to around 60–80 ng/dL *before* a TBI event happens to prevent further damage.

Now I'd like to share some additional nutrients that should be part of your TBI kit for ongoing support at home.

Omega-3 DHA/EPA

Essential fatty acids, especially DHA (docosahexaenoic acid), are the building blocks of neural membranes in the brain. EPA (eicosapentaenoic acid), another essential fatty acid, is also important for acute brain injury because of the way this omega-3 fatty acid is more of the signaling molecule that helps decrease inflammation in a gentle way.

Fish oil contains both of these fatty acids and has been shown to decrease the devastating effects of brain injury. In a University of London study, rats given DHA after spinal cord injury showed improved function of growth factors as well as decreased oxidative damage and lipid peroxidation, which is damage to the cell membranes. DHA also helps normalize levels of BDNF, a protein that is a growth factor for neurons.[10] Unfortunately, Americans are, in general, deficient in omega-3 fatty acids. Data from a National Health and Nutrition Examination (NHANE) survey conducted between 2003 and 2008 found that U.S. adults are not meeting recommended levels because they don't each enough wild-caught fish and or other foods high in omega-3 fatty acids, like nuts and seeds such as flaxseed, chia seeds, and walnuts.[11]

Pregnenolone

Pregnenolone is a broad-acting neuroprotective agent that has been found to be low in patients with a history of traumatic brain injuries. For military veterans with mild TBI, pregnenolone has been shown to help with insomnia, irritability, and hypervigilance—an advanced state of sensory sensitivity—by potently activating the gamma-aminobutyric acid (GABA) system, which is the brain's main inhibitory neurotransmitter. Basically, pregnenolone helps the nervous system calm down.[12]

Progesterone

Progesterone is a steroid hormone that exerts anti-inflammatory, anti-edema (swelling), neuroprotective, and neurogenic (growth) effects. Progesterone has been one of the most extensively studied treatments for TBI and has been shown to be effective in acute traumatic brain injuries in over two hundred studies.

I recommend taking progesterone only under the supervision of a medical professional trained in hormones so as not to cause disruption to the hormonal system.

Vitamin D and Progesterone

Applying the concept I have described in the previous chapter—that the intervention for brain injury should have multiple and broad mechanisms of action—I want to make you aware of research both in the lab and in human testing that demonstrates how combining progesterone with vitamin D works better than either substance alone.

In the lab, studies have shown that vitamin D with progesterone offered more protection to neurons.[13] Then, in an Iranian study of sixty patients with severe TBI, the first group had progesterone alone (patients were injected with 1 mg/kg of progesterone intramuscularly every twelve hours for five days and within twenty-four hours of the injury). The second group was given the same amount of progesterone plus 200 IU/kg of vitamin D once a day for five days. What this means is that a 150-pound person received 13,600 IU of vitamin D per day for five days. The third group received placebo injections and regular standard medical care for TBI. The results stated that 35 percent of the progesterone and vitamin D group had a "good recovery" compared with 15 percent in the control group and 25 percent in the progesterone-only group. The death rate in the control group was 40 percent, while the progesterone group was 25 percent and the progesterone and vitamin D group was only 10 percent. This study suggests that a combination approach is more effective for acute TBI than a single agent. This is the reason I recommend combining multiple overlapping substances in acute and chronic TBI treatment.

CDP-Choline (Citicoline) and Alpha-GPC

Part of correcting the integrity of damaged cell membranes includes reincorporating the components that make up those important pieces. Choline and specifically CDP-choline (citicoline), or another similar nutrient known as alpha-GPC (alpha-glycerylphosphorylcholine), are helpful for this structural component as well as helping feed into the acetylcholine system, thereby helping with memory and alertness. A large-scale meta-analysis of human subjects failed to show a large benefit of this one nutrient, but it did show some promise for enhancing cognition in chronic TBI.[14]

The dose I recommend is 500 mg twice daily up to 1,000 mg twice daily with food.

Ketone Bodies

Ketone bodies (betahydroxybutyrate, acetoacetate, and acetone) are carbon molecules produced from fatty acids and are an efficient fuel source for the brain. Ketone bodies are naturally produced by the liver from fatty acids.

Each morning when you wake up, you are in a mild state of ketosis if it's been twelve hours since your last meal. During periods of increased energy demands, such as after suffering a brain injury, the production of ketone bodies helps in the recovery. Ketone body production can be enhanced by either ingesting preformed ketone bodies such as betahydroxybutyrate or receiving a precursor such as MCT oil, which the liver then readily turns into more ketone bodies.

Another way to encourage production of ketone bodies is to eat a low-carbohydrate diet that's high in fat and moderate in protein. Fasting rapidly increases ketone body production naturally. Animal studies show that if an animal fasts for twenty-four hours after a moderate traumatic brain injury, the animal's ketone production will increase and circulate more ketone bodies that provide neuroprotection, decrease oxidative stress, maintain cognitive function, and improve mitochondrial function compared to the control group.

But who wants to undergo fasting that long for any reason? An easier but equally effective way to gain the benefits from ketone bodies is to ingest a source of fat that the injured body can rapidly convert into ketone bodies and circulate up to the brain.

Coconut oil is such a fat and contains a high percentage of shorter-chain fatty acids, called medium-chain triglycerides (MCTs), that the liver can convert into ketone bodies, which then cross into the brain and act as a fuel source and antioxidant. See chapters 7 and 8 on diet for more on this.[15]

Vitamins E and C

After a traumatic brain injury, there is a "rusting process" that happens where an increase in free radicals and reactive oxygen species leads to increased oxidative stress and further brain injury. This is called a "secondary injury." There have been several human TBI studies using the antioxidants vitamins C and E after a TBI to halt this secondary brain injury.

For instance, a study in Iran led by Dr. Razmkon in one hundred severe acute TBI patients demonstrated that using intravenous vitamin C (10,000 mg/day) reduced brain swelling. Vitamin E (via intramuscular injection at 400 IU/day) improved the outcome of those receiving vitamin C. In short, the antioxidant qualities of both vitamins C and E are essential to help the body heal.

Why do these two vitamins work so well together? It's because vitamin C is water soluble and vitamin E is fat soluble, so they are able to work on different areas both inside and outside the cell.[16]

Here are my dosing recommendations:

Vitamin C dosing. I recommend taking buffered vitamin C to "bowel tolerance," which means 1,000 mg every one to two hours until you begin to have loose stools or diarrhea, at which point you'll want to decrease the frequency of the dose. Alternatively, take a fat-soluble vitamin C—known as ascorbyl palmitate—at 1,000 mg twice daily for better absorption.

Vitamin E dosing. Vitamin E is part of a family comprising several varieties. When shopping for vitamin E, look closely for the mixed tocopherols with tocotrienols, as this is the vitamin E found in nature and is more effective. Much of the vitamin E sold today is d-alpha tocopherol, which has been shown to be harmful in several past studies. I also don't recommend the straight alpha-tocopherol form, which is readily available as well.

Studies have shown that using a "cocktail" of types of vitamin E results in little risk and much more benefit. Aim for around 375 mg of mixed tocopherols and 150 mg of mixed tocotrienols (one gel cap) twice daily.

A word of caution: vitamin E slightly increases the risk of bleeding, similar to baby aspirin. Check with your doctor before starting vitamin E.

Acetyl-L-Carnitine

Shortly after a traumatic brain injury, there is an energy deficit. Acetyl-L-carnitine essentially helps the mitochondria (the energy-producing powerhouse of the cell) produce more ATP (adenosine triphosphate), which is the energy currency of the body. In several animal studies, acetyl-L-carnitine has been clearly shown to reduce damage from TBI.[17]

In this study and other similar ones, researchers used 100 mg/kg, which would equate to around 6,800 mg of acetyl-L-carnitine for a 150-pound person, multiple times over the course of the day. While not harmful, such doses are not practical and are likely not needed, especially in combination with the other substances we have discussed.

Alpha-Lipoic Acid

Alpha-lipoic acid is a fat- and water-soluble antioxidant, meaning it can get into the brain and help both inside and outside the cells. Alpha-lipoic acid has proven to be effective at decreasing inflammation and reducing oxidative damage to cells. This nutrient has also been shown in studies to decrease glial scar formation (brain scarring after TBI) as well as support blood-brain barrier formation.[18]

The dosing recommendation is 300 mg twice daily.

L-Glutamine

In times of stress, the body has an increased need for certain amino acids such as glutamine, which is a fuel for enterocytes (small intestine cells). After a brain injury, the body is vulnerable to intestinal hyperpermeability (aka leaky gut). It is also common to have leaky gut after major traumatic events such as a severe burn or a major emotional stressor.

Many branched-chain amino acid products contain L-glutamine, so you don't have to buy an extra supplement.

LED Light

LED (light-emitting diode) light and cold-laser therapy have been shown to activate specific healing mechanisms when applied to the back of the neck and points on the head by carrying "light-infused" blood into the brain. Light therapy increases the function of the mitochondria, or energy-producing parts of the cell, thereby increasing cellular energy to a damaged brain as well as signaling release of nitric oxide, which in turn increases blood flow.[19]

The current research in animal models for acute traumatic brain injury is on lasers, which are called "cold lasers" because they do not cut the skin and are not hot at all. They are extremely bright, however, and can damage the retina if looked at directly. The LED light used for treating traumatic brain injury is so bright it is important to wear safety goggles or keep the light directly against the skin so as not to damage the eyes. Animal studies confirm what we see in other studies with nutrients like NAC and glutathione as discussed above: that laser therapy within twenty-four hours greatly reduces long-term problems from a TBI.[20,21]

A Plan of Action

You may be wondering if you need to take *all* of these supplements in order to heal from a traumatic brain injury. After all, that's a lot of different nutrients as well as capsules!

Here's a good way to get started. I would recommend taking the TBI first aid kit and adding a couple of specific nutrients, starting with fish oil and acetyl-L-carnitine. Then you could pick either vitamins C and E or alpha-lipoic acid as your main antioxidant source. These antioxidants have been shown to help prevent the long-term problems of brain injury. I'd like to see a head-to-head trial comparing vitamins C and E to alpha-lipoic acid to figure out what works better, but we do not have that research yet.

Use the acute TBI protocol for up to the first three months after a traumatic injury to the brain since this is considered the acute phase. You may not need it for more than a couple of weeks before you notice all of your symptoms resolve, however. The focus of treatment during this stage is on decreasing inflammation and oxidative damage, getting energy to the brain, and reducing any swelling that has taken place. After that, in addition to continuing to provide antioxidant support to the brain, there is a shift toward stimulating circuits in the brain that are underactive.

There is not one specific combination that works for everyone. The key is to make a plan that is manageable and sustainable both financially and physically for the person with the injury and their family. Think about dosing these nutrients based on what areas need the most improvement:

- If low energy is a concern, focus on acetyl-L-carnitine, MCT oil, and branched-chain amino acids.

- If pain and inflammation are more of an issue, increase curcumin and the antioxidants alpha lipoic acid and vitamins C and E.

Healing injuries will involve not just "taking things" like supplements but also involve "doing things" like exercise, changing your diet, and other therapies like cold laser, hyperbaric oxygen, meditation, or brain games.

Here's an outline of the optimal nutrients for traumatic brain injury:

Nutrient	Dosage	Notes
Vitamin D	10,000 IU acutely, then 10,000 IU daily for the next seven days, then 5,000 IU daily thereafter	Vitamin D levels should be checked as part of a lab workup as soon as possible, unless vitamin D status is known, and at least every three months thereafter until levels are replete, then every six to twelve months. Goal is 60–80 ng/dL.
Pregnenolone	50–100 mg twice daily	A neurosteroid used by both men and women for mild TBI. An NIH study of military veterans showed improvements in sleep and anxiety. It's best to check levels.

Nutrient	Dosage	Notes
Fish Oil	3,000 mg of omega-3 fatty acids daily	Omega-3s from fish oil (EPA/DHA) greater than 3,000 mg per day may increase the risk of a bleed. Ensure there is not a brain bleed by having a brain CT scan and evaluation by a doctor. Check with your doctor before going above 3,000 mg per day of combined EPA/DHA.
Vitamin E	375 mg of mixed tocopherols and 150 mg of mixed tocotrienols— 1 cap twice daily	This mix is important; you don't want just alpha-tocopherol. Vitamin E may slightly increase the risk of bleeding, similar to aspirin, so make sure to consult your doctor.
N-acetyl cysteine (NAC)	500 mg twice daily	NAC is a glutathione precursor as well as an antioxidant.
Vitamin C (buffered ascorbic acid)	1,000 mg twice daily	

Nutrient	Dosage	Notes
Curcumin	500 mg twice daily	Helps with swelling by opening up aquaporins.
Acetyl-L-carnitine	1,000 mg twice daily	Increases brain energy. May use more to gain more energy and to help with mood.
Alpha-lipoic acid	300 mg twice daily	Antioxidant (fat- and water-soluble), decreases glial scar formation.
Glutamine	2 grams twice daily	Helps the gut and protects against leaky gut due to brain injury.
MCT powder/oil	Ideally 3 tablespoons twice daily, but may use less if combined with exogenous ketones	Start with 1-teaspoon twice daily since larger doses can cause GI upset and diarrhea, especially if taken on an empty stomach. Try to find one that has a higher concentration of C:8 and C:10 fatty acids, as these will more readily be turned into ketone bodies.

Nutrient	Dosage	Notes
Exogenous ketones	1 packet twice daily Keto//OS (caffeine-free), KetonX, Kegenix	Start with a small amount like 1 teaspoon. Similar to MCT oil, exogenous ketones can cause upset to the stomach and cause diarrhea.
CDP-choline	500 mg–1,000 mg twice daily	

Exercise and Stimulating Activities

Besides taking optimal nutrients for traumatic brain injury like N-acetyl cysteine (NAC), curcumin, and pregnenolone or consuming "brain shakes" (see chapter 7 on diet), refraining from doing certain things is as logical and important—arguably, *more* important—component of recovery. It's important not to start doing strenuous exercises too soon after bodily injury. Just as important is to not tax the brain too soon after injury.

Just as athletes have to rest and recover before they are allowed to go back into the game, it's the same for those who've suffered a brain injury. Stimulating and taxing an already damaged brain may actually cause more damage and delay healing. That's why it's important for students to take breaks from studying or even delay entrance back into school after a concussion or brain injury. Excessive stimulation from TV, video games, and even reading can be mentally taxing. Work with your doctor on how quickly you can restart activities.

Often the rule of returning to play after one week is simply not enough time. I've worked with individuals, especially if they had multiple concussions, who needed several months or longer before they could return to playing their sport. If you have head pain or other symptoms return during or after exercising, then reduce the intensity by 25–50 percent and try again. Gradually increase the amount of time that you are concentrating or exercising. Increase by 25 percent per week, but it's okay to go slower if needed.

How do you know how much brain stimulation is too much? Take cues from your body: if you become tired or irritable after reading, doing homework, or even watching TV, then it's too much too soon. If you start having a headache after reading, then read for shorter amounts of time.

Chronic brain inflammation is like a smoldering fire that continues for hours. Just when you think the fire is all the way out, all it takes is a little dry brush or a piece of paper and the fire will ignite anew. Keep in mind that a chronic brain injury is challenged by excesses: excess inflammation from eating hydrogenated oils, excess in drinking alcohol, excess spikes in blood sugar, excess exercise, and excess stimulation from video games or even violent movies.

Have this mantra in mind: *The brain needs time to rest, heal, and recover.* Activities such as light reading and mild challenges such as crossword puzzles or brain teasers can be helpful, but not before one week, and then only if there isn't a recurrence of symptoms. As the brain gets stronger, try increasing the challenges by extending the reading time and the difficulty of the content. For students, see how much time elapses before you start having difficulty focusing, head-aches, or vision problems. The next time you study, go a few minutes less. You really don't want to push it, or you risk a delay in recovery time.

Avoid stimulating beverages like sodas, energy drinks, and coffee. These beverages can mask the truly weakened state of the brain because for a few hours you may feel alert and overdo it. I also recommend talking with your doctor about not taking stimulant medications, if at all possible. After sev-eral months you could resume these medications if needed, but you don't want to flog a dead horse, meaning that if the brain's neurons are not healing and are limping along, forcing them into action may stress them even more and impede heal-ing. It's better to take some of the approaches I've outlined in this book to help your figurative "wires" to reconnect.

Exercise is advisable after one week post-concussion. In general, exercise raises BDNF (brain-derived neurotrophic factor) and promotes healing. While this is true, a study look-ing at this topic demonstrated worsening of symptoms if started too soon after injury.[22] It's better to wait at least one week, lis-tening to your body the entire time. If your symptoms worsen during or after exercise, then it's too soon or too intense. Start with lower intensity and work up. If during exercising you begin to notice any significant fatigue, foggy-headedness, or headaches, it's time to back off and take a break.

A Concluding Thought

If a program such as the one outlined in this book were to be employed in a larger study, I'm confident we would see success, improving and even saving lives and helping a great many people.

Mainstream treatments from traditional medicine have been too focused in their mechanisms of action and sometimes too toxic in their effect. There are better treatments that are more effective than what is currently being done in medical practices around the country.

My hope is that by utilizing the tools outlined in this chapter, you will be armed to mitigate, if not eradicate, symptoms of long-term traumatic brain injury. The unfortunate truth is that most of those who are affected by traumatic brain injury are people who have been suffering for months and years with many of the symptoms they had thought would get better after a brief recovery time.

If that sounds like you, then know that things don't have to stay the same.

Notes

1. Hoffer ME, Balaban C, Slade MD et al. Amelioration of acute sequelae of blast induced mild traumatic brain injury by N-acetyl cysteine: a double-blind, placebo controlled study. *PLoS One.* 2013;8(1):e54163.

2. Dean O, Giorlando F, Berk M et al. N-acetylcysteine in psychiatry: current therapeutic evidence and potential mechanisms of action. *J Psych Neurosci.* 2011;36(2):78–86.

3. Laird MD, Sangeetha SR, Swift AEB et al. Curcumin attenuates cerebral edema following traumatic brain injury in mice: a possible role for aquaporin-4? *J Neurochem.* 2010;113(3):637–48.

4. Jeter CB, Hergenroeder GW, Ward NH et al. Human mild traumatic brain injury decreases circulating branched-chain amino acids and their metabolite levels. *J Neurotrauma.* 2013;30(8):671–79.

5. Eelen G, Verlinden L, van Camp M et al. The effects of 1alpha, 25-dihydroxyvitamin D3 on the expression of DNA replication genes. *J Bone Miner Res.* 2004;19:133–46.

6. Fernstrom. "Large neutral amino acids: dietary effects on brain neurochemistry and function." *Amino Acids.* 2013.

7. Kajta M, Makarewicz D, Ziemi'nska E et al. Neuroprotection by co-treatment and post-treating with calcitriol following the ischemic and excitotoxic insult in vivo and in vitro. *Neurochem Int.* 2009;55(5):265–74. doi: 10.1016/j.neuint.2009.03.010. Epub 2009 Mar 26.

8. Author manuscript. Having lower levels of vitamin D before injury sets you up to have worse damage and more difficulty healing. *Neurotherapeutics.* available in PMC 2011 Jan 1.

9. Hua F, Reiss JI, Tang H et al. Progesterone and low-dose vitamin D hormone treatment enhances sparing of mcmory following traumatic brain injury. *Horm Behav.* 2012;61(4):642–51.

10. Michael-Titus AT. Omega-3 fatty acids and neurological injury. *Prostaglandins Leukot Essent Fatty Acids.* 2007;77(5–6):295–300. Epub 2007 Nov 26. High levels of omega-3 fatty acids are recommended as soon as you can get going on them, but they are too messy to carry in your first aid kit and are not as stable as some of the other nutrients and risk rancidity. That is why I did not include them in the first aid kit. It is wise to have a good healthy level of omega-3s before brain injury as it has been shown in another animal study that deficient levels of omega-3s before a head injury leads to a poor outcome. So if you start out low and deficient in omega-3s, that will increase your vulnerability and slow recovery. See also Ying Z, Feng C, Agrawal R et al. Dietary omega-3 deficiency from gestation increases spinal cord vulnerability to traumatic brain injury–induced damage. *PLoS One.* 2012;7(12):e52998. doi: 10.1371/journal.pone.0052998. Epub 2012 Dec 28.

11. Papanikolaou Y, Brooks J, Reider C et al. U.S. adults are not meeting recommended levels for fish and omega-3 fatty acid intake: results of an analysis using observational data from NHANES 2003–2008. *Nutr J.* 2014;13:31.

12. Marx CE, Naylor JC, Kilts JD et al., eds. Translating biomarkers to therapeutics: overview and pilot investigations in Iraq and Afghanistan era veterans. *Translational Research in Traumatic Brain Injury.* Boca Raton FL: CRC Press/Taylor and Francis Group, 2016. Chapter 7.

13. Atif F, Sayeed I, Ishrat T et al. Progesterone with vitamin D affords better neuroprotection against excitotoxicity in cultured cortical neurons than progesterone alone. *Mol Med.* 2009;15:328–36.

14. Meshkini A, Meshkina M, Sadeghi-Bazargani H et al. Citicoline for traumatic brain injury: a systematic review and meta-analysis. J Inj Violence Res. 2017;9(1):41–50.

15. Davis LM, Pauly JR, Readnower RD et al. Fasting is neuroprotective following traumatic brain injury. *J Neurosci Res.* 2008;86(8):1812–22. doi: 10.1002/jnr.21628.

16. Razmkon A, Sadidi A, Sherafat-Kazemzadeh E et al. Administration of vitamin C and vitamin E in severe head injury: a randomized double-blind controlled trial. *Clin Neurosurg.* 2011;58:133–37.

17. Scafidi S, Racz J, Hazelton J et al. Neutoprotection by acetyl-L-carnitine after traumatic injury to the immature rat brain. *Dev Neurosci.* 2010;32(5–6):480–87. doi: 10.1159/000323178. Epub 2011 Jan 12.

18. Rocamonde B, Paradells S, Barcia C et al. Lipoic acid treatment after brain injury: study of the glial reaction. *Clin Dev Immunol.* 2013. Article ID 521939. See also: Toklu HZ, Hakan T, Biber N et al. The protective effect of alpha lipoic acid against traumatic brain injury in rats. *Free Radic Res.* 2009;43:658.

19. Naeser MA, Zafonte R, Krengel MH et al. Significant improvements in cognitive performance post-transcranial, red/near-infrared light-emitting diode

treatments in chronic, mild traumatic brain injury: open-protocol study. *J Neurotrauma*. 2014;31(11):1008–17. doi: 10.1089/neu.2013.3244. Epub 2014 May 8.

20. Oron A, Oron U, Streeter J et al. Low-level laser therapy applied transcranially to mice following traumatic brain injury significantly reduced long-term neurological deficits. J *Neurotrauma*. 2007;24(4):651–56.

21. Here are some references to research on lasers for acute TBI:

    a. Oron A, Oron U, Streeter J et al. Low-level laser therapy applied transcranially to mice following traumatic brain injury significantly reduces long-term neurological deficits. *J. Neurotrauma*. 2007;24(4):651–56.

    b. Khuman J, Zhang J, Park J et al. Low-level laser light therapy improves cognitive deficits and inhibits microglial activation after controlled cortical impact in mice. *J Neurotrauma*. 2012;29:408–17.

    c. Wu Q, Xuan W, Ando T et al. Low-level laser therapy for closed-head traumatic brain injury in mice: effect of different wavelengths. *Lasers Surg Med*. 2012;44:218–26.

    d. Xuan W, Vatansever F, Huang L et al. Transcranial low-level laser therapy improves neurological performance in traumatic brain injury in mice: effect of treatment repetition regimen. *PLoS One*. 2013;8:e53454.

I described in the example above using an LED light in order to quickly stimulate the healing process in Thomas. He could then see a provider who does laser therapy. Bioflexlaser.com has a list of providers, and many are familiar with concussion protocol.

22. Griesbach GS. Exercise after TBI: is it a double-edged sword? *PM R*. 2011;3(6 suppl 1):S4–72.

7

CAN WHAT YOU EAT HEAL YOUR BRAIN?

•••••••••••••••••••••••••••••••••••••

BRIGHT MINDS Principles

Inflammation: Inflammation in the gut can lead to inflammation in the brain. Optimizing nutrition and eating a diet that is high in anti-inflammatory foods will help lower brain inflammation.

Diabesity: The brain uses 20–30 percent of the calories in our diet. Injured brains have difficulty getting enough fuel, which leads to fatigue. Eating a diet high in refined carbohydrates and sugars not only hurts your brain now, but sets you up to have inflammation for the long term if you have a concussion.

•••••••••••••••••••••••••••••••••••••

Chris was at the end of his rope.

Two years after cracking his head on a sidewalk in a bike crash, he still struggled with daily headaches, crushing fatigue, and keeping his balance—all of which contributed to him losing his job as captain of a ferryboat that plied the San Juan Islands. His marriage was in divorce court because of the anger and rage he exhibited.

In the midst of this personal turmoil, Chris wasn't getting any better. After telling me that he had little money for treatment, he asked, "What are the one or two supplements I can take to heal my brain?" It was obvious that Chris wanted to get the most bang for his buck.

I told him that one of the most powerful treatments he could do for a brain injury was not to take a supplement but to change his diet. I recommended a version of the ketogenic diet, which is basically a low-carb, high-fat diet. Within one week, Chris noticed that he felt better, and his sleep improved. Within a month, as he faithfully stayed with his new way of eating, he experienced more energy, felt his depression lift, and started to lose the weight that he had gained in the past two years.

Among the types of treatments discussed in this book, your diet—the foods you eat and the beverages you drink—is foundational to your healing. Nothing else you do on a daily basis moves you closer to—or further from—healing and feeling better. I believe a modified version of the ketogenic diet is likely the most powerful, effective diet method for healing brain injury, which is why I'm using this chapter to introduce you to the rudiments of this eating plan.

In the following pages, I'll describe the practical side of actually following the ketogenic diet and then I'll answer some commonly asked questions regarding this diet plan.

Looking Back to History

Hippocrates, the "father of medicine," observed back in 500 BC that when patients with severe epilepsy fasted, their seizures stopped. This was a momentous discovery for ancient times and the first historical link between neurology and dietary interventions.

Then, in 1911, Parisian physicians also noted that fasting decreased the seizures of patients. In 1921, Dr. Rollin Woodyatt and Dr. Russell Wilder of the Mayo Clinic discerned that ketone bodies—three water-soluble molecules produced by the liver when fatty acids are broken down for energy—appeared in patients who were either in a starvation state or consuming a low-carb, high-fat diet. Dr. Wilder coined the term "ketogenic diet" and began treating epileptic patients accordingly.

What Dr. Wilder and his colleagues discovered is that ketone bodies seemed to have a healing effect on the brain as well as providing an alternative fuel source. They were aware that ketones had antioxidant effects and reduced oxidative damage in the brain.

Since that time, the traditional version of the ketogenic diet has always consisted of a high-fat diet with very low protein and very low carbohydrates. Around 80 to 90 percent of calories are from fat, and the rest comes from combined protein and carbohydrates, consisting mainly of cream, butter, eggs, and bacon. Vegetables are out because they are a source of carbohydrates, and most protein sources are out as well because the body can readily turn protein into glucose.

This may sound like an unhealthy way of eating, and I

thought so too when I first heard about the ketogenic diet. In fact, early research did not yield favorable results. Studies done, mostly with children, following the traditional version of the diet, left children with nutrient deficiencies and health problems. However, it's important to remember that these studies were based on an older version of the diet, with a very narrow scope of allowed food. The newer, modified version of the ketogenic diet, which I advocate, allows more protein, a little more carbohydrates in the form of green leafy vegetables, and is nutritionally high in many vitamins and minerals.

Kids, Epilepsy, and the Ketogenic Diet

I've found that most of the research performed on the ketogenic diet is focused on children because this diet has helped juvenile patients control their seizures.[1]

Neurologists found that putting children on a ketogenic diet not only ended their seizures, but also cured their epilepsy in several years. This allowed these children to live seizure-free lives and refrain from taking epilepsy-related medications.[2]

During the 1970s, researchers found that medium-chain triglycerides, or MCTs, were turned into ketone bodies by the liver. (MCTs are made up of medium-chain fatty acids commonly derived from coconut oil, palm oil, and dairy fats.) The liver can produce ketone bodies from other fat sources like long-chain monounsaturated fatty acids (found in olive oil) and polyunsaturated fatty acids (found in vegetable oils), but not as efficiently as medium-chain triglycerides. When these MCTs were added to the diet in place of some other fat, especially from dairy products, children were able to decrease the amount of fat and increase the amount of carbohydrates and protein they could eat.[3]

This was termed the *modified ketogenic diet* or MCT ketogenic diet because of the addition of medium-chain triglycerides. Since that time, multiple variants have been created to try and make the diet palatable while at the same time being therapeutic. In 2009, a study compared the classic ketogenic diet to the modified versions with MCT oil and found them equally effective for epilepsy.[4]

In recent years, the ketogenic diet has had a rebirth, even though you may not know that because it's been called many different names, including:

- Modified Atkins Diet
- Low Glycemic Index Therapy Diet
- Radcliffe Infirmary Diet
- Keto-Paleo Diet

Each diet plan shares the characteristic of using coconut oil—and its medium-chain triglycerides—to help the body preferentially shift to using ketones for fuel, even if some carbohydrates are consumed.

To get the most out of your carbohydrates, it's best to spend most of your carbohydrate "dollars" on vegetables and a few berries rather than grains or starchy vegetables like potatoes. You can consume small amounts of squash and cauliflower, as well as other green leafy vegetables in large quantities, and still maintain ketosis. That's because these veggies contain much more fiber and more complex carbohydrates, so they provide a kind of natural "slow release" mechanism and don't spike blood sugar levels.

The interesting side effect of the ketogenic diet is weight normalization: if done correctly, people who need to lose weight will lose it, and those who need to gain weight will gain it. What other diet is used by cancer patients who may be underweight as well as body builders and endurance athletes to gain muscle and lose weight if needed? There is growing research on the modified ketogenic diet's ability to rapidly normalize insulin resistance and help people with type 2 diabetes.

So how does the ketogenic diet help to heal brain injury?

The ketogenic diet is thought to be effective because of the healing effect of ketone bodies on the brain. In addition to its energy-stabilizing effects on the brain, the ketogenic diet also has neuroprotective effects. For openers, patients experience decreased oxidative stress, which is an imbalance between the production of free radicals and the ability of the body to detoxify their harmful effects through the body's antioxidant system. In fact, ketones themselves have antioxidant capacity.[5] (Please note this about the ketogenic diet: I'm not referring to ketoacidosis, which is a potentially life-threatening condition for type 1 diabetics. In this chapter, I'm discussing nutritional ketosis, whereby the body is not in a state of crisis but has simply shifted over from burning carbohydrates as its predominant fuel source to fats.)

In recent years, studies have shown that the ketogenic diet has helped a number of low-brain and energy-state conditions such as migraine headaches, Parkinson's disease, Alzheimer's disease, amyotrophic lateral sclerosis (ALS), cancer, stroke, mitochondrial disorders, depression, autism, and of course traumatic brain injury. A single common pathway of dysfunction for a number of neurological conditions is that a very hungry organ—the brain—is starving, and the ketogenic diet is one solution for replenishing it.[6]

This is an important point, because early in a traumatic brain injury, brain glucose levels rise and then drop below normal. Giving glucose—or high-sugar foods—to TBI patients certainly worsens outcomes.[7] A human study in which patients were fed a low-carbohydrate diet, but not a ketogenic diet, demonstrated they did have some ketone production compared to a control group fed a standard carbohydrate-rich diet.[8] A laboratory animal study where rats fasted after suffering a traumatic brain injury demonstrated that fasting for twenty-four hours after a TBI event was protective.[9] That said, we need more human research on the ketogenic diet for acute and chronic brain injury.

The Mechanism Behind the Ketogenic Diet

Our brains are hybrid organs that can burn either carbohydrates or fatty acids for fuel.

The brain is programmed to prefer glucose—which comes from carbohydrates—because the brain can break glucose down into energy quickly. If the brain does not have abundant glucose, however, it will switch from using glucose as its primary fuel source to using fatty acids that come from dairy products, coconut oil, fish oil, and so forth.

One benefit of using fatty acids for brain fuel is that the energy is steady. Also, burning fats produces a higher total amount of energy than burning carbs. The biochemistry is complex, but in the end, it boils down to this: *Burning fat for fuel produces approximately three times as many calories—gram for gram—as glucose.*

This may be why many on the ketogenic diet have improved energy and mental clarity and report they have less need for sleep. This was certainly the case for me when I tried it—after an adjustment phase, that is.

I've found that when I've been on the modified ketogenic diet for about four to six weeks, my body adapts to a point where I need about one hour less sleep per night. For a father of three young and energetic kids with a busy work schedule, I knew I wasn't getting enough sleep until I found out that being on the modified ketogenic diet meant I could cheat the clock.

Two reasons I went on the modified ketogenic diet in the first place were because:

1. I often recommended this diet plan to patients and didn't want to recommend something that was too difficult for me to do.

2. I tend to have low blood sugar and thus a low energy state. When I started the modified ketogenic diet, I had rock-solid blood sugar and energy levels.

A ketogenic diet may help those with Alzheimer's disease because of the energy's effects on the brain. One of the problems with Alzheimer's disease is that the glucose transporters—the proteins that transport glucose across cell membranes—are damaged, and therefore glucose does not get into the brain very well.[10] The brain is literally starving!

Ketone bodies, however, can be transported across cell membranes because their transporters are not damaged. It's like they use a backdoor energy pathway into the brain, which is why this diet works well in healing those with traumatic brain injury; since an injured brain is in a hypo-metabolic state, meaning it's in need of energy but unable to get it.[11]

If you eat a higher-carbohydrate diet, which most of us do, the brain will use those carbs for fuel first and not readily make fatty acids into ketones. Your brain, however, is used to getting into this mild ketogenic state while you sleep. Each morning, when you wake up, you're usually in a mild fasting state in which your body turns fatty acids to ketones in the liver and send them up to the brain as a fuel source. This is why it's important to start your day in "low-carb mode"—if you are trying to attain a state of ketosis. Your brain and body will be more "open" to the process.

If you continue to eat a lower-carbohydrate diet, you will continue to burn ketones as well as stored-up glycogen (glucose stores) as fuel. After about three days, when your body has depleted its supply of glycogen, there is an increase in ketone production as the body shifts over to more full-time nutritional ketosis. Adding healthy fats to the "menu," especially MCT oil, further enhances that process. In short, eating a lower-carbohydrate, moderate-protein, higher-healthy-fat diet provides the most energy-rich environment in which you can heal from a traumatic brain injury.

Now that you know some of the "why," I'll talk about how a modified version of the ketogenic diet might be just the ticket for you or a loved one dealing with a traumatic brain injury and how to get started.

Trying on the Ketogenic Diet for Size

I believe the modified ketogenic diet is the path to success. Yes, it is a somewhat time-intensive and complicated plan, but it's certainly attainable, and studies have shown it is the most therapeutic diet for brain injury.

So, maybe you're all pumped up and ready to start this life-improving process! But changing one's diet is hard, so I'm recommending that you start slowly and in phases. That way, change is more feasible. Remember, progress—not perfection—is the goal.

Here's a road map you can follow:

1. See your doctor before you start. Always consult with your doctor before making any major dietary change. Once both of you decide on a plan of action, ask to be checked for nutrient deficiencies such as low iron, zinc, copper, and selenium, which, if low, may make the transition into the modified ketogenic diet more difficult. Also ask to have your thyroid checked as well as an electrocardiogram (EKG) to make sure your heart rhythms are healthy. You don't want to have a prolonged QT interval, which can cause irregular heart rhythms. These irregular heart rhythms can cause fainting, seizures or even death. This is probably due to the electrolyte changes that can happen when getting started on a ketogenic diet. Heart rhythm disorders can happen during periods of starvation, but that shouldn't be a problem on the ketogenic diet, because you eat to satiety while consuming meats, vegetables, and fats. However, some people on certain medications may see an increase in the QT interval, which is why you want to know prior to starting the ketogenic diet. If you do have a prolonged QT interval, it does not necessarily mean you can't try the ketogenic diet, but either correcting it or monitoring your heart while on it will be important.

Many people like to have their health markers checked before and during the diet to see how cholesterol and inflammation levels change. Know that they typically and predictably go down.

One medication to be cautious with is Topamax, an anti-seizure pharmaceutical that has the potential to increase kidney stones. I had a patient who started the ketogenic diet and was on Topamax for partial complex seizures. She was being hit with involuntary convulsions almost daily, but when she started the ketogenic diet, her seizures were significantly reduced, and working with her neurologist, she was able to stop taking Topamax. I cautioned her to stay well hydrated, especially during the first phases of the diet, so that she wouldn't develop kidney stones or other difficulties.

2. Ease in. You don't have to go overboard on changing your diet. *Any* improvement in diet will help your brain. The list below provides a framework to help you set up for success. These steps are based on where you are with your dietary habits, how much time you can invest, and how damaged your brain is, even though you can start at any point along the scale. The steps build on themselves, so if you start out with the goal of cutting out gluten, it's assumed you're making sure you consume protein at each meal and are cutting out sugar.

So here are my suggested steps for easing into the ketogenic diet:

- Cut out sugar for one week to break the addictive nature of sugar on your taste buds and the habit of eating sugary and sweet foods for comfort, stimulation, or reward. Then eat only fruit as dessert after that.

- Eat protein at every meal and snack. This means chicken, beef, eggs, or a protein shake at breakfast. For a snack, nuts, hummus, or a protein bar are excellent sources.

- Eat vegetables a minimum of twice daily. Examples would be green leafy vegetables like lettuce, spinach, kale, or broccoli. Think about what grows above the ground (leafy vegetables) vs. what grows below the ground (like potatoes). Ideally, half of what's on your plate should be green leafy vegetables.

- Cut out gluten-containing grains for at least one month. Then challenge your new status quo by reintroducing gluten in its simplest forms to see if it's a problem. Gluten irritates everyone's gut a little bit; some are more sensitive than others.[12] Clinically, I have seen that gluten is one of the most fatigue-producing grains, and when gluten is cut out of the diet, energy improves for many people.

- Add healthy fats such as avocados, coconut oil, olives, olive oil, nuts, and seeds to each meal.

- Decrease your carbohydrate intake and increase the healthy fats and proteins. Many people feel substantial benefit just from cutting out gluten and going low on carbohydrates and higher on protein, healthy fats, and vegetables. To see what this might look like on a practical level, see the Modified Ketogenic Diet Meal Plan that I've provided later in this chapter.

- Add in MCT oil. When you do so, your diet now contains all the major pieces of the modified ketogenic diet. You can check to see if you are in ketosis with blood-testing strips or through breath or urine testing. (See more information on the ketogenic diet below.)

And please, remember that all stages of diet should include adequate water intake.

If you aren't quite ready for the modified ketogenic diet, that's okay; you can take comfort in the fact that you may not need this diet to heal. Know that making any improvement to your diet will improve your brain health.

I saw a twenty-one-year-old male patient, who I'll call Randy, who was having episodic brain fogginess and low energy after a concussion. His injury happened during football practice a year earlier.

Following my consultation, Randy was compliant with my recommendations to make adjustments in his diet. He ate protein with each meal and was gluten-free and dairy-free the rest of the time. (In my experience, the two most common food intolerances are gluten and dairy.)

Randy noticed significant improvements in his energy level and a decrease in brain fog. Secondarily, he noticed that when he minimized the consumption of sugary foods like raspberry jam, chocolate chip cookies, apple pie, and vanilla bean ice cream, he noticed additional benefits and reported that he felt "amazing, better than I have felt in years."

Randy didn't need to go a step further into the modified ketogenic diet because he noticed improvements by simply cutting out gluten and dairy. When he cut back on sugar, his health took another notch up in the right direction. I told Randy that he may still need to go on to a modified ketogenic diet if he plateaus at some point and that it wouldn't be a bad idea to add some medium-chain triglyceride oil to his diet to increase ketone production.

3. Know that correcting elevated blood sugar is key for brain healing. If you have metabolic concerns such as prediabetes or metabolic syndrome (a combination of high blood sugar, high blood pressure, elevated cholesterol, and excess fat around the middle), your body and brain will have more inflammation and less energy for your brain cells. Less energy will slow down your healing.

If you have elevated blood sugar, then eating low carbohydrates is critical. A blood test such as a hemoglobin A1C will help determine if you have elevated blood glucose levels. A great way to reduce elevated blood sugar levels is by cutting out gluten because it naturally cuts down on many carbs. Be cautious not to replace all of the gluten-containing grains with gluten-free processed junk food like cookies and desserts, however.

4. Don't jump too fast. I've said that changing your diet is both an accessible and an important treatment you can apply, and I've also said there's a difference between "important" and "easy."

For some people, changing their diet is one of the most difficult things they could do. For many, it's almost like changing a part of yourself when you eschew foods that you've grown up with. But if changing what you eat improves your ability to live your life to the fullest, isn't it worth it to work on changing and redefining yourself?

Because making a change to the diet can be overwhelming, my patients tend to go into "all or nothing" mode. I think that makes it much harder for them! The key to making a big change to your diet, like any formidable task, is *preparation*—both mental and physical. Start with stages, and advance to the next level only when you think you're ready. I would urge you to consider making this diet change within the next month and start with two or three days a week. Here's a checklist that you can follow:

❏ **Don't start immediately!** It's okay to set a date when starting a new way of eating, which can be in a week or a month from now. This also gives you time to mentally prepare for the task at hand. When you're ready, shop for all of the things you're going to eat for breakfast, lunch, dinner, and snacks.

❏ **Reframe your thinking.** Remember that carbs are usually just filler anyway; the flavor is in the toppings, the vegetables, the sauces, the meats, the fats. And remember, too, that it takes time to get used to new habits. For example, after living in a gluten-free family for many years, I've gotten used to bunless burgers and actually prefer them to regular burgers because the bun isn't in the way of the flavor of the good stuff in the middle.

❏ **If you're out and about, be prepared by bringing snacks to tide you over until you get home.** For instance, if you're doing the ketogenic diet, pack a baggie with macadamia nuts or walnuts. Take along MCT oil or MCT oil powder in a small bottle or MCT oil capsules in a ziplock bag.

❑ **When you're out to eat, make good choices.**
It's possible to find something that fits in your diet.
Here are a few specific tips:

- Chipotle and other fast-casual restaurants: order a salad bowl with meat, grilled vegetables, salsa (not corn), and double guacamole.

- Fast-food hamburger places: order a bunless burger, hold the French fries and ketchup (sugar). To accompany the patty, ask for extra mustard, extra mayo, extra pickles, a little onion, and any other low-sugar condiment instead.

- Thai food: if you have a sensitivity to gluten or dairy, Thai food can be a challenge for following a modified ketogenic diet because of the common use of sugar. Ask the chef to prepare dishes without added sugar. Good options are a coconut curry, Tom Kha Gai (coconut milk soup), or stir-fried vegetables and meat without rice or noodles.

- Italian food: good options are antipasto, meat sauce without the spaghetti noodles, or a fatty steak such as a rib eye or a piece of fish like salmon. You can add some butter to the side vegetables of asparagus, broccoli, or spinach.

- Gyro stands: you can order the gyro salad with shawarma meat instead of gyro meat, as the gyro meat is often loaded with flour or bread. Don't forget the olives for good fats and extra flavor.

149

- Don't forget that many restaurants have options where you can request meat and vegetables without the potatoes, rice, and bread or toast, etc.

❑ **Eat more fat than you think you need.** This means adding fat to each meal vs. just eating a meal that has fat in it such as meat or eggs.

- Make sure you cook those eggs in at least 1 to 2 tablespoons of coconut oil or butter.

- Add some avocado to every meal.

- Add mayonnaise, oils, butter, or fats to each meal.

The First Few Days

After starting the modified ketogenic diet, you can expect during the first few days to feel like you are fasting or have low blood sugar.

This is an important time to take it very easy and not do a lot of exercising. Drink extra water, because ketones have a mild diuretic effect. Add extra salt to your food, because it's easy for the body to lose water and salt. Improving the retention of water and salt helps with dehydration and muscle cramps.

Once the glycogen or stored glucose is gone, your body switches into a fat-burning or ketosis mode. You should start to feel better at this point. Be aware that it may take several weeks to feel significant energy improvements when you are more fully "keto-adapted," as it were. For some who have significant nutrient deficiencies, this may take longer.

One time, I had a patient who had, on her own, started a ketogenic diet. It took her months for her to start feeling better, and she couldn't figure out why. When I had her nutrient levels checked, she was severely anemic. Once we got her iron levels up, she felt significantly better.

When I tried the modified ketogenic diet, I failed at my first attempt. I didn't understand that the feeling of low blood sugar was temporary and would change after three days. I figured that since I had a fast metabolism, then maybe I just couldn't do a low-carb diet.

Yes, my blood sugar was low, but after several weeks, I snapped out of it and felt clearer and sharper than I had in years. One telling sign that something was different was at bedtime. Normally, as my wife, Drie, and I turn out the lights, she tends to be chatty. Try as I might, I usually fall asleep right away. On the third day of the modified ketogenic diet, however, I won Husband of the Year honors for talking her to sleep that night.

What was happening was that my body switched over to burning fats for fuel instead of carbohydrates. Taking extra MCT oil certainly helped, as did drinking a lot of water, salting my food liberally, and taking potassium and magnesium supplements. Ketosis tends to deplete your electrolytes since it's a diuretic, so drinking more than you think you need to is important. If you feel hungry, you're probably not eating enough fat.

Endurance athletes and those who want to burn fatty acids for fuel will actually prepare their bodies for a race by eating a low-carb, higher-fat diet a couple weeks before a race to prime their systems to burn fats. By eating this way, endurance athletes successfully increase the efficiency of their bodies to use fat for fuel, reduce fatigue, and increase endurance. Long-distance athletes also carbo-load on the eve of the race, eating lots of pasta and breads so that they will experience a surge of power from the carbohydrates.

I'm a runner who's completed a few triathlons over the years, so I have firsthand knowledge of what happens when you put certain types of foods in your body in the weeks and days leading up to a big race. When I followed the ketogenic diet, I didn't get tired as I usually did during the heat of competition. I felt I could keep going and not get the lactic acid buildup that I would normally get.

Traditions, Habits, and the Need for Reinterpretation

Food supplies have changed over time, but our bodies haven't changed nearly as much.

Or, said another way, our bodies weren't designed to handle large amounts of carbohydrates, which are staples of the standard American diet. Thanks to the advent of modern agriculture, we have easy access to wheat grains and starchy crops like corn and potatoes. Back at the beginning of time, though, our forebears were hunter/gatherers who were often in a ketogenic state because of all the different plants and vegetables they ate, as well as from the meat of the animals they captured and killed.

Fast forward to today, when we have so much, as well as freedom to make food choices without much guidance as to what our bodies need. Food is more than fuel today. Unfortunately, we use food as comfort, telling ourselves that "I deserve this treat" or that "I'm lovin' it" as we step into our favorite fast-food restaurant.

Food should be enjoyed and celebrated, and it's okay to have a piece of cake on your birthday. But what will get you is that sweet muffin with your coffee each morning, that foot-long sandwich for lunch, those four slices of pizza for dinner, and that generous helping of German chocolate cake for dessert every night.

So, what's the best diet for optimal brain health? Is such a diet practical? Will one be able to eat out? Or will it get weird?

The following is a ketogenic diet meal plan that is not only practical but one that could change lives, including yours or that of a loved one dealing with a traumatic brain injury. Without further ado, here's a plan to get you started:

The Modified Ketogenic Diet Meal Plan

Breakfast

Scramble two to four eggs with 1–2 tablespoons of onions, ½ to 1 cup of spinach, a bit of mushrooms and olives, cooked in 1–2 tablespoons of coconut oil. Optionally, you can add half to a whole avocado. Pour 1 tablespoon of MCT oil on the eggs, or take it by the spoonful.

Other meals you can prepare for breakfast:

- Antipasti, which is one of my go-to breakfasts also because I can make it and sneak out of the house while the kids are still asleep. Here's a recipe I follow: 3 ounces of salami (nitrate-free), ¼ cup olives, 1 avocado, some sprouts or other salad, and 1 tablespoon of MCT oil on the olives and avocado. Sprinkle the avocado with salt and pepper.

- I also like a keto smoothie: 1–2 tablespoons MCT oil, coconut cream or milk, or unsweetened almond milk, 1–3 teaspoons of unsweetened cocoa powder, 10–15 drops of stevia, 20 grams of low-carb protein powder, a handful of greens like kale or spinach, and 1 or 2 ice cubes.

- You can also eat dinner leftovers or prepare a salad with chicken or pork sausage using a ranch dressing, but make sure it's sugar-free. Add a half-cup of olives and one tablespoon of MCT oil.

Morning Snack

Celery or red pepper sticks with sugar-free ranch dressing, fortified with extra olive oil or MCT oil.

Lunch

A large salad with 4 ounces of chicken, 1 tablespoon of olive oil dressing, 1 avocado, ½ tablespoon of sunflower seeds, 1–2 sliced radishes, 4–5 olives, plus 1 tablespoon MCT oil on the salad or by the spoonful.

Other meals you can prepare for lunch:

- Salmon salad using canned salmon, pickles, mayonnaise, mustard, pepper, dill weed, squeeze of lemon juice over salad, or, even better, use cabbage leaves to scoop it up. Plus 1 tablespoon MCT oil mixed in or by the spoonful.

- Leftover grilled or roasted meat with salad and dressing. Add MCT oil, olives, avocado, radishes, and other greens.

Afternoon Snack

Eat 10 macadamia nuts or cashew nuts.

Dinner

Grilled meat or fish (4–5 ounces), steamed or sautéed green leafy vegetables like kale, chard, and/or spinach (in coconut oil), zucchini, steamed or grilled asparagus, or some other low-carb veggie. Add 1–2 tablespoons MCT oil on the salad and veggies after they are cooked or by the spoonful.

Other meals you can prepare for dinner:

- Prepackaged low-carb Thai curry such as Marion's Kitchen Thai Red Curry with 4–5 ounces of chicken, beef, or pork and green veggies such as kale, chard, mushrooms, and onions. Add extra coconut cream or coconut milk. Serve over cauliflower rice.

Cauliflower rice is made by chopping the cauliflower finely in a food processor (until the pieces are about the size of rice grains), squeezing out some of its water, and then sautéing the cauliflower in olive oil until it's hot and softened. Add an extra tablespoon of MCT oil.

- Chorizo or other sausage with grilled veggies such as asparagus, or roasted broccoli, which is prepared by mixing generous amounts of broccoli and olive oil and baking at 350°F for 10–15 minutes or until the florets are cooked but still slightly crunchy, flipping the broccoli halfway through. Add salt afterward, because the salt pulls out water from the broccoli and it will become dehydrated instead of caramelizing.

- Stir-fry chicken, beef, or pork (4–5 ounces) with mushrooms, kale, green beans, and onions. Serve with cauliflower rice or salad.

- Steak salad, which is a mixture of grilled steak, lettuce, cabbage, green onion, homemade guacamole, and chimichurri sauce.

Evening Snack (Optional)

Mix ½ cup coconut cream, 1–3 teaspoons unsweetened cocoa powder, 1 tablespoon cashew or almond butter, ½ tablespoon MCT oil, and 5–10 drops of stevia. Stir vigorously by hand, then put the bowl in the freezer and let freeze for 10–20 minutes, and then enjoy.

Or you can make a pudding by mixing 2 cups of coconut cream or coconut milk with ¼ bar of unsweetened dark chocolate and letting it melt. Stir in ¼ to ½ cup of a sweetener like Swerve, xylitol, or erythritol. Then whisk 1 tablespoon of gelatin into the mixture. Stir in 3 tablespoons of MCT oil. Pour into ramekins and refrigerate for 1 hour. Optional: sprinkle cocoa nibs or a couple raspberries over the pudding.

FAQ

These are some common questions I hear in my practice:

Are there risks with the ketogenic diet?

The ketogenic diet is complicated and does have some risks if not followed correctly. Then again, all diets involve some type of inherent risk and take planning to follow. At the same time, the ketogenic diet promises healing and is a unique treatment for a host of neurological conditions. In my estimation and experience, the ketogenic diet is well worth considering if you or a loved one has had a traumatic brain injury.

Some of the controversy around the ketogenic diet, such as the claims that it's nutritionally deficient, comes from research done more than twenty years ago on children who were fed nutritionally deficient dietary "fat" shakes that were missing key vitamins and minerals. The newer modified ketogenic diet has been dramatically improved upon and does not have these same problems, thanks to the consumption of more vegetables and protein sources like meats and some nuts.

Here's a short list of conditions where the ketogenic diet is probably not a good idea:

- Kidney stones
- Active gallstones
- Impaired liver function
- Gastric bypass surgery
- Decreased gastrointestinal motility
- Abdominal tumors
- History of kidney failure
- Pregnancy or lactating
- Pancreatitis
- Eating disorders
- Fat metabolism disorders
- Certain metabolic conditions and genetic conditions
- Certain heart conditions

In short, talk with your doctor before starting any new type of dietary intervention.

Will the ketogenic diet raise my cholesterol levels?

Yes, it will raise them, but it's not bad news.

Of course, everyone worries that cholesterol will increase the risk of heart attacks and strokes. But the *American Journal of Clinical Nutrition* published an analysis in 2010 clearly stating that saturated fat in the diet is not associated with an increased risk of coronary heart disease or cardiovascular disease.[13] This study clearly showed that lower-carbohydrate, higher-fat diets had no long-term adverse effects on cholesterol levels.

This type of diet tends to increase both the HDL (good) and LDL (bad) cholesterol levels, though it also predictably and consistently lowers the triglyceride levels, which changes the "bad" LDL from the small, dense kind to the large, buoyant, and more protective kind.

One twelve-month study compared high-fat, higher-protein diets vs. low-fat diets. Those who went on the low-carb diets lost more weight and lost weight more easily and more quickly than those on the low-fat diets.[14] The study also found that cholesterol levels were not as correlated to heart disease as once thought.

Do I need to take extra supplements on the ketogenic diet?

Yes, especially during the transition phase, which is the first three days and then the first three to six weeks until you are "keto-adapted." Long-term supplementation is helpful even after this stage.

Being in ketosis and eating a low-carbohydrate diet causes a diuretic effect whereby salt is excreted. If you have a tendency toward low blood pressure already, you will need to watch out for this. Be heavy-handed with the sea salt, even if this is more salt than you think you need. You should consume higher than normal amounts of water, especially during the first three days.

Potassium supplements may be helpful as well. I found that taking around 500 mg of potassium helped me when I was feeling dehydrated during the first few days on a ketogenic diet.

Magnesium works as a natural mind- and muscle-relaxer that can help with leg cramps and sleep. Given that, magnesium is best taken at night. People used to get magnesium from stream-fed water or and spring water, which can be replicated by drinking natural "mineral water" such as San Pellegrino.

Here are some amounts to shoot for:

- **Salt:** 1–2 grams daily, and be sure you're generous with the saltshaker. You can also consume olives as well.

- **Potassium**: 300–500 mg daily, but check with your doctor about this as some medications do cause potassium reabsorption, and you don't want your levels going too high.

- **Magnesium glycinate**: 300–1,000 mg daily. Effervescent or powdered magnesium, such as the Natural Calm brand, is a highly absorbed form of magnesium made into a drink. By mixing with almost-boiling water, the magnesium ions are freed and become more absorbable. (Magnesium glycinate doesn't cause loose stools as readily as other forms such as magnesium oxide or magnesium citrate.)

A Concluding Thought

Because prescription drugs are easier to take, the traditional ketogenic diet is rarely used anymore as a first-line therapy for seizure or other disorders. But it's been my experience that the modified ketogenic diet (or other "simple" dietary choices you can make) can help your body achieve the desired and healthy state of ketosis without feeling underfed and deprived. To date, the research is more favorable for children with brain injury using the modified ketogenic diet than it is for adults. But I've seen patients of all ages find the ketogenic diet to be highly energizing and useful in helping them focus more than any other type of diet.

That's not to say that this way of eating is for everyone. Personally, I found the ketogenic diet most helpful for the first three to six months for brain function. For many cycling it in and out for periods of time works better than staying on it for the long term. People whose brains function best on moderate protein and moderate carbohydrate diets—often athletes or individuals with a high metabolism—will probably want to stay the course, but if you or someone you care for has had a traumatic brain injury, then you have everything to gain by trying out the modified ketogenic diet.

Notes

1.   Levy RG, Cooper PN, Giri P. Ketogenic diet and other dietary treatments for epilepsy. *Cochrane Database Syst Rev.* 2012.

2.   Vining E, Freeman JM, Ballaban-Gil K et al. A multicenter study of the efficacy of the ketogenic diet. *Arch. Neurol.* 1998;55(11):1433–37.

3.   Wheless, James W. History of the ketogenic diet. *Epilepsia.* 2008;49(8):3–5.

4.   Neal EG, Chaffe H, Schwartz RH et al. A randomized trial of classical and medium-chain triglyceride ketogenic diets in the treatment of childhood epilepsy. *Epilepsia.* 2009;50(5):1109–17. doi: 10.1111/j.

5.   Haces ML, Hernández-Fonseca K, Medina-Campos ON et al. Antioxidant capacity contributes to protection of ketone bodies against oxidative damage induced during hypoglycemic conditions. *Exp Neurol.* 2008;211(1):85–96. doi: 10.1016/j.

6.   Stafstrom CE, Rho JM. The ketogenic diet as a treatment paradigm for diverse neurological disorders. *Front Pharmacol.* 2012;3:59.

7.   Robertson CS, Goodman JC, Narayan RK et al. The effect of glucose administration on carbohydrate metabolism after head injury. *J Neurosurg.* 1991;74:43–50.

8.   Ritter AM, Robertson CS, Goodman JC et al. Evaluation of carbohydrate-free diet for patients with severe head injury. *J Neurotrauma.* 1996;13:473–85.

9.   Davis LM, Pauly JR, Readnower RD et al. Fasting is neuroprotective following traumatic brain injury. *J Neurosci Res*. 2008;86(8):1812–22.

10. Simpson IA, Chundu KR, Davies-Hill T et al. Decreased glucose transport 3 immunoreactivity in the performant pathway terminal zone. *Annals of Neurol*. 1994;35(5):546–51.

11. Giza CC, Hovda DA. The neurometabolic cascade of concussion. *J Ath Train*. 2001;36(3):228–35.

12. Junker Y, Zeissig S, Kim SJ et al. Wheat amylase trypsin inhibitors drive intestinal inflammation via activation of toll-like receptor 4. *J Exp Med*. 2012;209(13):2395–408. doi: 10.1084/jem.20102660.

13. Siri-Tarino PW, Sun Q, Hu FB et al. Meta-analysis of prospective cohort studies evaluating the association of saturated fat with cardiovascular disease. *Amer J Clin Nutr*. 2010;91(3):535–46.

14. Gardner CD, Kiazand A, Alhassan S et al. Comparison of the Atkins, Zone, Ornish, and LEARN diets for change in weight and related risk factors among overweight premenopausal women: a randomized trial. *JAMA*. 2007;297(9):969–77.

8

CORRECTING STRUCTURAL INTEGRITY

• •

BRIGHT MINDS Principles

Blood flow: A hit to the head or even whiplash can cause damage. There can be narrowing of the supporting structures and restriction of blood flow or even the flow of spinal fluid, causing severe headaches, balance problems, fatigue, and depression.

Head trauma: The head is heavy and sits atop the vulnerable neck, and damage to the supporting structures (bones, connective, tissue and fascia) can cause long-term problems, such as pain, headaches, balance problems, and dizziness.

• •

Everyone knows that dizziness can be debilitating.

Imagine walking down a hallway like you're aboard a lurching boat or feeling off-balance or nauseous because of black-and-white-striped patterns on the carpet. Dizziness and balance issues caused by damage to the brain are problematic and troubling to anyone dealing with this affliction.

Beatrice was a highly successful executive until she experienced a serious brain injury. She had been drinking and was playfully wrestling with her boyfriend in the living room when they fell over together and she hit her head on the corner of a coffee table. The next day, after she woke up, Beatrice got out of bed and felt like she was listing to one side. She attributed her inability to stand up straight to the drinking she'd done the previous evening. But day after day, the symptoms of feeling like she was trying to maintain her balance on the deck of a moving sailboat persisted.

By the time Beatrice came to see me, she had tried a bunch of different treatments and medications, but nothing helped. I suggested several initial treatments that lessened her symptoms, but she still wasn't able to function normally and had to go on disability.

I encouraged her to see a chiropractor with additional training in functional neurology. I was aware that doctors trained in functional neurology can help "reset" the nervous system after it has been disrupted by a brain injury or another stressor. I explained that one of the leading practitioners is Dr. Ted Carrick of the renowned Carrick Institute in Cape Canaveral, where he is one of the professors teaching advanced training for techniques in neurology.

While Dr. Carrick is one of the pioneers of this approach, he is not alone. There are many others taking a functional approach to health care, and among them are medical physicians, naturopathic physicians, osteopathic physicians, and optometrists. I like how Dr. David Burns, a Seattle chiropractor and naturopathic physician, describes functional neurology as "not specific to chiropractic, naturopathic or medical. It is a way of thinking, evaluating and treating humankind. What I look for is how various brain systems or regions are performing. This assessment is partly to do with symptoms being experienced, partly to do with how the level of function compares to others, and partly how one side of the patient compares to the other (e.g., reflexes)."

Dr. Burns compares the brain to a bunch of muscles, and he considers himself to be a personal trainer for the brain and nervous system. He helps identify weaknesses, and then works to strengthen them.

I told Beatrice that I had many patients benefit from this approach, and it helped them with their dizziness. If you've gone through a long bout of debilitating symptoms like hers, then I recommend that you check into seeing an expert in functional neurology.

Correcting the structural integrity of your body and brain is a key for healing from a TBI. Think of these physical medicine techniques as making sure the "house" has a stable foundation before building the walls, windows, and roof. This can be done by seeing one of the medical specialists I'll talk about in this chapter.

Your practitioner needs to take an inventory of the physical issues that relate to different areas of the brain. Here's a comprehensive, but not complete, list to consider when it comes to coordination and balance problems:

- Light sensitivity
- Dizziness
- Muscle weakness
- Difficulty speaking
- Headaches
- Muscle tension
- Tingling or numbness
- Insomnia
- Arm/shoulder pain
- Low back pain
- Sciatica
- Hip/knee/foot pain
- Body tremors

Once your medical practitioner understands what you're dealing with, you can discuss a treatment plan. Here's an explanation of several approaches that I recommend:

Functional Neurology

I've already mentioned functional neurology, which focuses on rebalancing the neurological system through the use of specific movements and exercises that often involve the eyes. There isn't much of the traditional "adjustment" techniques where the bones are aligned, although there may be some of that. The idea is to bring an out-of-balance nervous system back into balance.

What does functional neurology generally look like? Typically, there is an initial intensive assessment and treatment phase that may last for five days all the way up to two weeks, during which you're asked to come in and see the doctor and his or her team every day. After that, there are maintenance exercises and follow-up visits, as needed. For patients having to come from out of town, this form of intensive treatment is best since they can return for maintenance periodically.

Upper Cervical Chiropractic or Atlas Orthogonal

The first vertebra in the spine is called the atlas, and it's upon this atlas that the skull sits and allows the spinal cord to pass up through a hole in the bottom of the skull, which is called the foramen magnum.

Think about how vulnerable this area is. If the first vertebra were, for some reason—such as whiplash or concussion—to move out of its rightful place and push into that space, a portion of the spinal cord's circulation of cerebrospinal fluid (CSF) would be cut off. This can cause a host of harmful symptoms that include vertigo, headache, tinnitus, facial pain, otalgia, dysphagia, and pain from weak muscles, dizziness, and impaired vision.[1,2] This may also increase the pressure in the brain and cause the brain to herniate out of the skull down through the foramen magnum when you're sitting or standing in an upright position.

Things other than TBI can cause cranial cervical syndrome, such as birth defects and severe arthritis, but the condition due to brain injury is much more common than previously realized.

Dr. Scott Rosa, a chiropractor who has been doing research in this area,[3] believes that an MRI done in an upright position is beneficial in assessing the problem. One of Dr. Rosa's main points—and he has research to back this up—is that in certain positions, the blockage happens, but at other times—such as when you lie down on your back—it doesn't. So, let me ask this obvious question: How is an MRI usually taken? Lying down, of course, which raises another question: How is an MRI going to capture this pathological phenomenon?

An upright MRI mimics what is happening in real life. Gravity can move the vertebrae and the skull out of place and block the flow of the cerebrospinal fluid, which causes pressure inside the brain to increase. Sometimes the pressure builds so much that parts of the brain are forced into the foramen magnum, which is a condition known as cerebellar ectopia.[4]

Dr. Rosa has documented, through the use of an upright MRI (by sitting in an MRI machine), that impingement before and after an adjustment of this vertebra improves and opens up the flow of CSF for those who have this vertebra out of place. This is an important piece of information to evaluate when you consider this form of treatment. (See the illustrations on the next page.)

It's not necessary to do an upright MRI to prove this point, but it's nice to know that this diagnostic tool is available. An

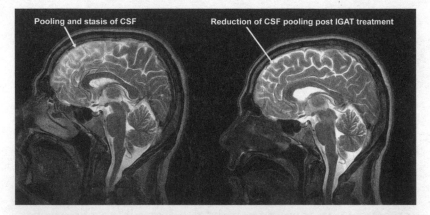

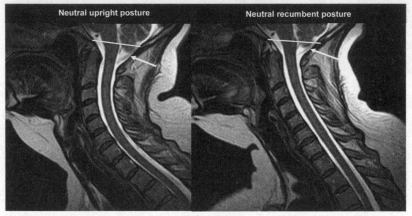

The first pair of scans show side views of the brain. On the left, impingement due to an out of alignment cervical vertebrae is decreasing CSF (cerebral spinal fluid flow) in the brain. On the right, after a cervical adjustment the CSF is flowing normally. © Dr. Scott Rosa

The second pair of scans show that when the patient is laying down in the MRI scanner (left) there is no herniation of the cerebellum down through the foramen magnum, but when the patient is upright in a special MRI scanner (right) the weight of gravity pulls the cerebellum down through the space (foramen magnum) where it shouldn't be, creating symptoms such as headache. The scan argues for upright MRIs to reveal pathology. © Dr. Scott Rosa upper cervical chiropractor or a NUCCA (National Upper Cervical Chiropractic Association) chiropractor can assess and correct your atlas without the use of an upright MRI. It's important that you find a healthcare provider who is well-trained in this area.

A typical treatment begins with a thorough examination of the position of the atlas (the C1 vertebra). X-rays of the upper cervical vertebrae and skull also need to be taken, and a specialized neurological examination should be performed. Only then will the chiropractor do an adjustment, using a subtle technique that doesn't involve any "cracking."

Craniosacral Therapy

Craniosacral therapy, a gentle, hands-on approach to release tensions deep in the body to relieve pain and dysfunction, was developed by Dr. John Upledger, an osteopathic physician. This subtle method does a terrific job of releasing tension specifically in the skull and spinal cord, hence its name "craniosacral therapy."

The goal is to release restrictions in the soft tissues that surround the central nervous system by moving the bones of the skull and working with the movements of CSF between the brain and the skull, down the spinal cord into the sacrum, which is the large bone at the base of the spine that makes up part of the hip girdle. Freeing up areas that may be blocked or trapped due to trauma to the head improves this flow of CSF.

A typical treatment entails usually a mood-enhancing setting like a quiet room with a massage table where the practitioner uses an extremely light touch—about the weight of a nickel—on different parts of the head and back. This very light touch, surprisingly, can cause significant changes in the body.

One young man who had had concussions while playing ice hockey found that after just one session of craniosacral therapy, his headaches went from five days per week to two days per week. Typically, patients report that after several sessions they begin to feel relief. I have found that craniosacral therapy is consistently helpful for TBI, which is why I think it is a therapy worth considering as part of your treatment plan.

Neurocranial Restructuring

Another technique worth considering is neurocranial restructuring, which also has a goal of realigning the bones of the skull to free up tensions. This technique involves insertion of tiny balloons into the nasal passages and then inflating them to adjust the cranial bones. Neurocranial restructuring is especially helpful if there is frontal damage either from blows to the face or forehead as well as chronic sinus problems.

I first learned about this method while in school when a fellow classmate of mine, Hillary Lampers, who had been studying with the developer of this method, Dr. Dean Howell, gave a demonstration to the class. Guess who volunteered to be a guinea pig?

When tiny balloons were inserted into my nose and inflated, I was surprised to hear a "crack," which realigned my sphenoid bone. But it wasn't painful at all. I have witnessed many patients with chronic sinus problems benefit from this method when receiving therapy from Dr. Lampers and others trained in this method. Unfortunately, not many are trained to do this technique, but it is my hope that it will become more widely available.

Choosing a Direction

When it comes to healing from a brain injury and correcting structural integrity, one of the key pieces of the puzzle is to make sure early on that something serious is not happening. If there is a blockage of cerebrospinal flow or the body is literally out of place, just about any method that is employed will be less effective.

The good news, though, is that correcting structural integrity is usually complementary to other therapies outlined in this book and does not interfere with, but rather balances, them. As far as deciding which direction to go, you may have the decision made for you depending on what practitioners are in your area. Upper cervical chiropractors and craniosacral therapists are probably the most widespread and numerous, but if you happen to live near a location where there are functional chiropractors, then I would suggest seeking them out.

Here are some resources to help you find a provider who can help correct structural integrity:

- To find a functional neurology chiropractor, check out the American Chiropractic Neurology Board website at acnb.org/DoctorLocator.aspx

- To find an upper cervical chiropractor or NUCCA chiropractor, check out the National Upper Cervical

Chiropractic Association website at www.nucca.org/
directory/

- To find someone well-versed in craniosacral therapy, visit the American CranioSacral Therapy Association website at www.acsta.org/

- To find someone who practices neurocranial restructuring, visit the NCR Doctors website at www.ncrdoctors.com/

I must admit, when I began treating patients with TBI at the Amen Clinics, sometimes I was at a loss about what to do when they weren't getting better. I went back to the principles I had learned in naturopathic medical school, especially a philosophy known as the "therapeutic order," where drugs and surgery are used as a last resort and other methods employed first. The therapeutic order posits that we should treat a patient using the least force first. The principles, in order:

1. **Identify and address the obstacles to healing to establish the foundation for optimal health**
2. **Stimulate the body's self-healing mechanisms**
3. **Strengthen weakened systems**
4. **Restore proper structural integrity**
5. **Use natural treatments**
6. **Use pharmaceutical treatments**
7. **Use high-force (invasive) interventions**

Correcting structural integrity was something I overlooked at one time, but now I'm a believer after witnessing great results in patients who add this structural piece to their treatment plan. Since adding the component of aligning the bones, the neurological systems of many more patients have been helped who otherwise wouldn't have.

Be sure to seek out one of the physical medicine providers listed in this chapter to give you the greatest chance of recovery.

Notes

1. www.merckmanuals.com/home/brain,-spinal-cord,-and-nerve-disorders/craniocervical-junction-disorders/craniocervical-junction-disorders.

2. Terrahe K. The cervico-cranial syndrome in the practice of the otorhinolaryngologist. *Laryngol Rhinol Otol (Stuttg)*. 1985;64(6):292–99.

3. Rosa S, Baird JW. The craniocervical junction: observations regarding the relationship between misalignment, obstruction of cerebrospinal fluid flow, cerebellar tonsillar ectopia, and image-guided correction. In Smith FW, Dworkin JS, eds. *The Craniocervical Syndrome and MRI*. London, Melville, New York: Karger, 2015.

4. Flanagan MF. The role of the craniocervical junction in craniospinal hydrodynamics and neurodegenerative conditions. *Neurol Res Int*. 2015;2015:794829.

9

BRAIN TRAINING: FROM MEDITATION TO NEUROFEEDBACK

∙∙∙∙∙∙∙∙∙∙∙∙∙∙∙∙∙∙∙∙∙∙∙∙∙∙∙∙∙∙∙∙∙∙∙∙∙∙

BRIGHT MINDS Principles

Blood flow: Meditation and brain training improves blood flow to the parts of the brain that need it most, like the attention and memory centers.[1]

Mental health: "Brain exercise" listed in this chapter will not only help decrease stress, but also improve the focus and resilience of your brain.

∙∙∙∙∙∙∙∙∙∙∙∙∙∙∙∙∙∙∙∙∙∙∙∙∙∙∙∙∙∙∙∙∙∙∙∙∙∙

As a society, our ability to focus has diminished significantly every decade or so.

I would harbor a guess that the advent of smartphones and their excessive use, by teenagers and adults alike, have decreased our ability to focus by 5 to 10 percent. Speaking from personal experience, I find it easy to get lost in the number of interesting articles and snippets of information on the Internet and often forget why I originally logged on.

Perhaps you can plead guilty as well. But think about it: If you wanted to weaken your ability to sustain attention, what would you do? What would be the best and surest way to decrease your ability to concentrate and weaken the frontal lobe?

Well, if you want your brain to be less organized, less thoughtful, more impulsive, and more unable to process emotions, then watch more TV, spend more time on your phone, and retire to the basement to play video games until dawn.

Anyone who is a parent or who has worked at a daycare center can tell you that after a few hours of being around children below the age of ten, you will feel scatterbrained, because children have a way of wanting your attention constantly. My wife, Drie, who tends to our children each day, sometimes complains about having "mom brain."

So what is "mom brain," or "parent brain" for that matter? In simple terms, it's a condition where neuroplasticity has gone awry. In such a scenario, your brain becomes less focused on one specific task and finishing that task to completion. I am not insinuating that having children retrains your brain in a negative way, but what I'm trying to point out is that watching kids all day—like playing hours of video games, watching mind-numbing sitcoms or lame movies, or wasting an evening on Facebook—is like eating dessert all the time and consuming no nutritious food.

Whatever you *feed* your brain is a way of telling it what you want it to do or how you want your brain to perform. What you want to do is feed your brain in a way that strengthens it and trains it to be sharp, quick, and agile. It's like exercising: we work out to condition our body and perform optimally. So, too, must we exercise the brain. We should be proactive in giving our brain a bit of a workout to strengthen it and keep it functioning at its highest level. Some simple ways to do that are to read a book, write in a journal, go on a long walk, work out in the gym, or meditate, which is probably one of the most effective and lowest-tech ways of brain training.

With that as our baseline, what I want to do in this chapter is focus on using neurofeedback and certain brain games to train the brain.

Starting at the Beginning

Before I explain more about neurofeedback and brain games, let's review the importance of the prefrontal cortex, which is the part of the brain that's most often damaged in traumatic brain injury. Specific problems associated with a damaged prefrontal cortex include the following:

- Difficulty in paying attention
- Difficulty in decision-making
- Difficulty in restraining impulse control
- Difficulty in reading
- Difficulty in planning ahead

When something is not right with the prefrontal cortex, one will have difficulty following directions. They will be given a list of steps to complete and only remember the first or second items and not the third, fourth, or fifth on the list. These are both signs that all is not right with the prefrontal cortex.

You may think that a person exhibiting these behaviors is just absentminded or disorganized, or that these are symptoms that someone with ADHD would have. And you'd be right. But it's been my experience that too many brain injuries are often dismissed or mislabeled as attention deficit hyperactivity disorder. This happens frequently in my office where a patient will come in complaining of ADHD symptoms that were "acquired" later in life. Sometimes acquired ADHD is from drugs, alcohol, or other toxins, but more often attention-deficit symptoms stem from a brain injury.

As a way of background, true ADHD is genetically inherited and starts in childhood and stays with people all their lives, which helps to differentiate it from other causes of attention problems. Many children and adults with ADHD, however, will take more risks because of the nature of the disorder, which makes them more susceptible to brain injuries. Of course, repeated head injuries makes their ADHD worse. It's a vicious cycle.

If you feel some of the symptoms I listed above, or you would simply like to strengthen your focus, impulsiveness, or problem-solving ability, then consider some of the treatments in this chapter, especially meditation and neurofeedback, which can help the emotional component of problems caused by TBI such as anxiety, depression, and irritability.

Let's start with some simple and effective forms of brain training that you can begin right away. After I've introduced these methods, I'll turn to several high-tech options to strengthen the brain, such as brain games and neurofeedback.

Meditation

Meditation is, in some ways, the perfect and most tried-and-true brain training on the planet. Meditation has been around in some form since humans have been around. Over thousands of years, meditation has developed into different sophisticated systems with traditions and religion surrounding it. I view meditation more like an exercise of the mind and not religious at all, even though many spiritual communities have adopted this practice because it's a useful tool for becoming more present and aware of God in their lives.

Meditation is simply paying attention to your thoughts. Jon Kabat-Zinn, a famous researcher of meditation and creator of the program known as Mindfulness Based Stress Reduction, which is taught in hospitals and clinics around the world, describes meditation as "paying attention on purpose in the present moment, non-judgmentally." When you think about it that way, it doesn't seem like there is much to it; after all, most of the time nothing much is happening in the present moment and your thoughts are usually rather mundane. But just try it sometime. It doesn't take more than a second before the engines of the mind turn on and start churning out thoughts, worries, and to-do lists pulling you in a different direction. Then try to bring yourself back to the present and label that thought "thinking." The brain's thinking is almost like another physiological process, and the brain is like a muscle that can be strengthened like you strengthen your arms, legs, and heart.

When you hear the word *meditation*, you may conjure up a picture of a yogi sitting cross-legged on a mountaintop with a completely blank and serene mind. I can tell you that's not necessarily an accurate picture. When I'm meditating, there's a lot going on and my thoughts are pinging all over the place. It's like I'm trying to build a birdhouse and mosquitoes keep biting and distracting me. My goal in those situations is not to become a feast for the mosquitoes so I swat them away, but my focus returns back to building the birdhouse.

When it comes to meditation, the birdhouse is your breath or your heartbeat. When a thought comes in, you want to label it "thought," which is the equivalent of swatting the mosquito and then bringing the focus back to your breath (the birdhouse). What's important—and something I learned recently—is that what actually strengthens the mind is not the absence of thoughts, but capturing the distracted mind and bringing it back to focus on the breath, for example. I call that a series of bicep curls for the mind: bringing the thought back, bringing the thought back, and bringing the thought back.

Meditation aims to strengthen the frontal lobe, the part of the brain involved in focus, while simultaneously allowing emotions to release their grip. By focusing on one thing—or closely watching your thoughts—you put some distance between the mind and the emotions.

There are different types of meditation, and all are helpful. Spiritual meditation, for example, focuses on God's love. There are types of "moving meditation" where you walk slowly and focus on each footstep. "Chanting meditation" is where a prayer or phrase is sung or chanted. The type of meditation that I've found useful is "mindfulness meditation," which focuses on one thing such as breathing but allows the free flow of thoughts and ideas.

The goal is to be an objective observer. Once you have a thought, notice it, and gently bring back your awareness to the present moment. There's no judgment. You don't look to the past or worry about the future. It's not about solving problems or coming to any epic revelation. It's just about being fully awake—in your life and in the moment.

The mental effort necessary for mindfulness meditation is actually one of the hardest things I have ever done in my life. It certainly seemed nearly impossible at first. But it made sense that it was so hard, because it wasn't something I was used to doing. I did get better with practice.

One of my longtime friends, Dan, has been a serious meditator for many years. Back in 2000, just before the New Year, he dragged me to a three-day silent meditation retreat, which seemed like a good idea at the time. Just hours into the retreat, I couldn't imagine sitting on a cushion for another fifteen minutes without uttering a single word, let alone another two and a half days! What had I gotten myself into?

I somehow survived the first day and broke up the sitting

meditation with walking meditation and something called "mindful eating," which helped pass the time. I can't say that I really ever "got it," but meditation is not something you "get" anyway. Meditation is something you have to practice and do, and in the doing you get the benefit. Meditation is kind of like brushing your teeth: it's something good to do every day, a way to polish your true self, which you see every time you look in the mirror.

Meditation does a body good. Even at my silent retreat nearly twenty years ago, I'll admit that I felt peaceful and focused at the end of three days—as well as sore in my knees and back.

That said, I couldn't wait to get back to civilization. But those three days of silence helped me realize that I truly wanted to meet my life partner, because I was ready and lonely. Shortly thereafter I met Drie, the woman who is now my wife. I'm not saying a three-day silent meditation retreat will help you find the woman or man of your dreams, but sitting in silence does help you focus better on what you truly want and what is important in life.

I've found that meditating with a group is much easier. I recommend taking a class called Mindfulness-Based Stress Reduction, which is a great introduction to meditation. If you can find a class near you, then I recommend trying one. They even have an online course, which can be found at www.umassmed.edu/cfm/mindfulness-based-programs/mbsr-courses/mbsr-online/.

You can also do a search for Mindfulness-Based Stress

Reduction, designed originally by Jon Kabat-Zinn at the University of Massachusetts Medical Center.

The Benefits of Meditation

Mindfulness or meditation may sound impossible to someone who has had a brain injury.

Sitting still and focusing? It's not going to happen.

If you're thinking that way, then you need to know there is thorough research demonstrating that meditation can help with brain injury. I'm aware of a landmark study that greatly changed the way meditation is viewed in the traditional medical community and opened the doors for this practice to be a respected part of medical practice for those facing changes in brain and immune function.[2] Some of the studies specific to brain injury were done by Dr. Ruthann Knechel Johansen, author of *Listening in the Silence, Seeing in the Dark: Reconstructing Life After Brain Injury*, and specifically deal with the long-term fatigue associated with brain injury.

For instance, stroke or TBI patients, one year out from the injury, showed significant improvements on mental fatigue just from meditating. Meditators in the study were assessed and found that attention, speed, and memory were also better.[3] Early research in 2003 from a pilot study found that patients with mild to moderate brain injuries who participated in a twelve-week meditation program and then were tested one year after their injury showed improvements in quality-of-life scores. Interestingly, patients also found more meaning and value in life.[4]

This 2003 study also showed alterations in brain activity

measured through electrical brain activity as well as improvements in immune function. The left side of the frontal lobe, which is more associated with positive emotion, was also more activated.

Meditation Exercise

If you're ready to get started with meditation, begin by sitting quietly, either in a chair or in a cross-legged posture on a cushion. Try to sit as comfortably as possible. Start by focusing on your breathing. Don't try to alter it or control it. Just pay attention to each inhalation and exhalation. Once your breathing becomes relaxed and regular, begin a "body scan," which means focusing on each part of your body, one part at a time. For example, you can start with your left foot. Press your foot against the ground and try to feel all the sensations you can. Then do the same with your right foot. As you move your attention up your legs, feel your pelvis and sitting bones supporting you.

Next, move up through your belly and into your chest. Make sure you feel your belly and chest moving in and out with each breath. Next, feel your back and your neck, and then each of your arms and hands.

Can you feel your face? You may not think you can, but try to allow all of the tension to leave your face. After you've completed this task, allow your entire body to be as relaxed as possible. Finish by feeling grounded and relaxed in your sitting position, continuing to pay attention to your breath, which is also known as "centering." Some choose to chant or softly say, "Sa Ta Na Ma," while others say "OM." For those religiously inclined, you can mediate on the God of Love.

There are a couple of meditation apps that I recommend: Insight Timer and HeadSpace. There are also neurofeedback devices that you wear on your head such as the Muse that can help you meditate by giving you feedback about when you are in a meditative state or not. The military is studying this device on soldiers.

High-Tech Brain Exercise: Neurofeedback and Brain Games

Now I'd like to move on to several sophisticated ways to balance and strengthen the brain, which generally is known as neurofeedback.

You may have heard of biofeedback (also called biological feedback). A classic example of biofeedback is measuring the heart rate and then doing something to lower the heart rate, which is associated with being more relaxed and less stressed. Neurofeedback is similar to biofeedback in that it's measuring the body, but what makes neurofeedback different is the way it measures brain waves or the electrical activity of the brain via an electroencephalogram or EEG.

When parts of the brain are overactive, one may experience anxiety, agitation, and insomnia. In the case of brain injury, parts of the brain such as the prefrontal cortex are often underactive, and this can be detected with neurofeedback equipment. When neurofeedback is employed, the brain's electrical activity is measured, and then training can be used to set it back to its normal and healthy state.

Neurofeedback has been used for at least fifty years. Some of the original research done on cats showed that after neurofeedback training, their brains were more stable and resistant to the effects of rocket fuel that would normally cause seizures and eventually death. NASA began training their astronauts using neurofeedback, and to this day, it's still part of their astronaut training program.[5]

Children benefit from neurofeedback as well. Multiple trials with children comparing stimulants such as Ritalin to neurofeedback repeatedly show that neurofeedback was equivalent to stimulant medication and the results are just as long lasting.[6] In fact, neurofeedback restructures the brain in a positive way, something Ritalin just doesn't do. And after one year, the results of neurofeedback still held for those individuals who had undergone the training.[7] According to the American College of Pediatrics guidelines published in 2012 regarding treating patients with ADHD, neurofeedback has a Level 1 recommendation alongside stimulant medications and behavioral therapy. Unfortunately, you won't find neurofeedback listed in their recommendations today, and it's because of the costs and time associated with doing twenty to forty sessions, or more, which a fairly standard approach for traditional cortical surface neurofeedback is training.

Furthermore, it is important to understand that the practice of neurofeedback has evolved dramatically over the last forty years. In the early years, neurofeedback was practiced as a symptom-based approach, meaning success was determined by symptom reduction, and system-driven protocols are vulnerable to numerous problems that would include poor outcomes.[8]

Today, it is common to do neurofeedback with the guidance of qEEG (quantitative electroencephalography)—a more advanced measure of electrical activity in the brain. Although there are clinicians who continue to practice neurofeedback (NFB) in its archaic form, qEEG-guided neurofeedback has developed into a standard approach. EEG-guided neurofeedback eliminates the dangers of a symptom-based model, and with excellent precision, normalizes areas of the brain that are identified as poorly regulated in the clinical presentation analyzed in a qEEG evaluation. A baseline qEEG assessment is taken before neurofeedback begins and another assessment is done after treatment.

The profession of applied neuroscience, however, offers even more advanced neurofeedback approaches, such as full-cap training. This approach is referred to as LORETA: low resolution electromagnetic brain tomography in 3-D. In this advanced approach, the client is prepped to wear a nineteen-sensor cap that trains the brain to regulate problems such as autism, ADHD, depression, anxiety, sleep disorders, traumatic brain injury, seizure disorders, post-traumatic stress disorder (PTSD), and learning problems. This advanced approach can also provide peak performance training for athletes and those working in high-performance positions. Advanced professional software can provide the client with more in-depth analysis and training to attenuate a variety of clinical complaints both at the cortical and subcortical regions of the brain.

Guide to Neurofeedback for TBI

For those with serious TBI, two dozen sessions or so of neurofeedback may be worth it, because there's a growing body of evidence that neurofeedback is effective for TBI. In 2013, the *Annals of Clinical Psychiatry* reviewed the literature on neurofeedback and found that all studies indicated benefits with some being significant and others demonstrating mild improvements.[9]

I have found this to be the case in my practice. I've had plenty of patients experience life-changing improvement while others have had minimal benefit.

As discussed, not all neurofeedback systems are created equally, so it's helpful to know a little bit about what type of neurofeedback you are shopping for. Here is a review of some notable neurofeedback options:

1. qEEG LORETA neurofeedback. In the hands of highly trained professionals, this is the best system to use. It is typically offered by psychologists. Many sensors are placed on the cranium. Before-and-after assessments are done.

2. Traditional EEG neurofeedback. This system is much simpler than the more sophisticated qEEG LORETA neurofeedback system, but with a skilled provider, traditional EEG neurofeedback can be highly effective and has a history of robust research to back up its use. This type of neurofeedback is typically provided by psychologists.

3. Brand-name neurofeedback. These prepackaged devices are effective but are limited because they have preset programs that train the brain in specific areas. Some brands to look for include NeurOptimal, Brain State, and EEG Info (aka Othmer Method).

While psychologists typically have the most training in neurofeedback, I've met a number of highly skilled and trained professionals including registered nurses, therapists, and naturopathic doctors who have been well trained in neurofeedback. It's important, however, to ensure that a trained neurofeedback clinician is nationally board qualified. The best way to determine this is to contact BCIA (Biofeedback Certification International Alliance) at bcia.org. This organization sets high standards for neurofeedback qualifications and will provide referrals upon request.

When investigating your options, it's helpful to ask about the type of neurofeedback system they use and how much experience they have with traumatic brain injury treatment. It's also important to know whether their neurofeedback equipment is FDA approved and at a professional grade. What this means is that the clinician is using neurofeedback software that includes the capacity to change the inhibit and reward bands when necessary versus the limitations of other neurofeedback equipment that can only offer preset training programs.

Whatever system is used, neurofeedback is a powerful and effective therapy for traumatic brain injury and attentional problems.

Brain Training

If you want your brain to be stronger at memorizing, you should play challenging games like bridge, spend some time doing a Sudoku puzzle, or try learning another language. In other words, do something to stimulate those brain cells. Just like exercising our bodies was not something we thought of as necessary one hundred years ago since half the country's citizens worked on farms, many people today don't think they need to "exercise" their brains. But science has confirmed this is not true.

I've found it interesting that conventional wisdom says that retirement age is a time to relax and stop working. Now research is showing a link between a stop in work and the time when memory problems start to be noticed. I have seen this pattern frequently. I can't tell you the number of patients who come to see me six months, one year, and two years after retirement complaining about memory loss and not being as mentally quick as before. This is because their brains are shutting down parts that aren't being used.

This doesn't have to be the case. I believe you can and should keep your brain sharp and active after retirement and up until the very end of life, if you take good care of it. By continuing to learn new things and challenging your brain, you can actually become mentally stronger. The best way to maintain the strength of the neuronal circuits is to constantly test them with new information and a variety of problems that need solving. If you don't use it, you lose it. This is why students forget calculus or facts from history class one week, one month, or one year later. When we let our brain get complacent by not actively engaging it, it will lose its edge. It's why there is the stereotype of the senior citizen who is mentally slow and forgetful.

I must point out, though, that there are several benefits to an aging brain, so it's not all bad news. Dr. Elkhonon Goldberg, in his popular book *The Wisdom Paradox: How Your Mind Can Grow Stronger as Your Brain Grows Older*, wrote that as more information is gained and self-reflection and insight is gained, observations around us can become more nuanced. This, he said, is essentially wisdom.

One definition of wisdom is being able to pick out patterns and make decisions based on accumulated information. There is certainly a slowing in processing speed, but it takes time to sort through all that information that has been acquired over a lifetime. There is also less quickness as far as recall, and learning new information is harder and something that really should be worked on to continue to strengthen the brain and not let old habits and laziness take over.

The other benefit to aging is that there tends to be better emotional regulation compared with younger adults. Older adults tend to react less to negative situations, ignore irrelevant negative stimuli better, and remember relatively more positive than negative information.[10]

I view all these things as a positive. We can't expect to remember everything, and in some ways it's helpful to forget certain facts that are not likely to be relevant to our lives, and focus on the positive instead.

My counsel is that if you are struggling in a particular area, then find a fun way to improve things. If you feel like you're having trouble focusing, then turn off Instagram and flip on a meditation app like Insight Timer and do five minutes of meditation to help with concentration, or play some focusing games on mybrainfitlife.com.

If it's a poor memory you want to improve, then maybe there's a language you've always wanted to learn. Our clinic manager Mayra speaks Spanish, so I like to dust off my high school Spanish when she teaches me new words and teases me when I pronounce them incorrectly. The point is the areas that are weakest need the most work. It's like going to the gym: if you have weak legs but strong biceps, then you need to work out your legs more and your biceps less.

Doing math is a great workout for the brain. If calculus was something you really enjoyed, then find some easy calculus problems on the Internet and "spark" those neurons all over again. If you're a World War II buff, read a book about the rise of Nazism or the planning behind D-day. When engaging in small talk with friends, ask interesting questions to spark new lines of conversation and elicit new bits of information from your friends. Curiosity is good, and look at the quest to learn something new as a way to keep the brain vibrant.

High-Tech Brain Training

Neurofeedback is a more sophisticated type of high-tech brain training, but there are simpler strategies of brain training available. In fact, there are types of brain training that target specific areas of the brain—areas that need support.

How do you know what works when it comes to training neurons to fire? And will the right areas of the brain be targeted? I'm pleased to report that there are tons of simple games available on mobile devices that do a great job stimulating the right areas of the brain. For example, a brain-training program called Captain's Log Mind Power Builder helped increase executive functioning—brain processes that help people plan, organize, and complete tasks—six months after the training period.[11]

Cogmed, a brain-training program available only on a desktop or laptop computer, includes before-and-after testing and weekly check-ins with a coach (usually a psychologist) who's available to help you. BrainHQ or CogniFit are robust programs as well. I also like the following programs for their ease of use and for their effectiveness, even though they don't have as much research behind them:

- Lumosity
- Elevate One
- MyBrainFitLife

MyBrainFitLife, designed by Amen Clinics, includes a validated and standardized cognitive test that's similar to a battery of tests that we use to measure all patients admitted to Amen Clinics. (Be sure to check out www.mybrainfitlife.com.)

Cognitive testing should be done prior to trying any of these brain-training exercises to help identify areas to focus on for brain training. These brain games can also help with emotional recognition in others, something that's sometimes lost after a TBI. Look at brain training like you do regular exercise: it's something you want to schedule and plan for. All you need is five to fifteen minutes a day to make solid progress.

In general, a brain game should be hard but not so hard that you don't want to continue or are ready to give up. Look at it as a worthwhile challenge that you'll only get better at.

Because the brain is like a muscle, weak areas can be strengthened. All it takes is repeated practice.

I saw how practice pays off when my daughter, Adailia, started playing basketball at five years old. I watched her throw the ball as hard as she could toward the hoop in an arc only to fall short three feet every time. No matter how hard she tried, she couldn't get the ball to the hoop.

Naturally, Adailia wanted to give up, but when she would see her big brother practice his shooting, she would try again.

It took her a while, but her persistence paid off one spring day when she launched the ball and swoosh! Adailia squealed in delight. After that, she made basket after basket without a miss. What she did in the beginning was to continue trying even though there were no results.

This is true for your brain as well. If you're not persistent in trying to get better or get stronger, you're always going to remain weak physically and mentally. It's going to take time and practice, but don't look at this as a painful time—it can be fun learning new things and feeling mentally fitter.

Remind yourself that brain games really are games. If you're competitive like I am, it's a hoot trying to beat your last score, especially if playing the brain game is going to improve your memory. Wouldn't it be great to remember someone's name or stay alert during long meetings or in the classroom? And you can accomplish this by playing games!

Some Things to Remember

Brain training and neurofeedback are best undertaken during chronic stages of brain injury and *not* during the acute phases. Nutrient and hormonal deficiencies should also be identified prior to the commencement of any rigorous brain-training program. Brain training is most effective as a part II strategy to *strengthen* a weak brain, not to fix a broken brain.

Here's what you should do today: download the Insight Timer or HeadSpace meditation apps or simply sit quietly and follow your breath for five minutes. Then you can try brain training by challenging your memory and focus with a brain game app, or you can go through a more sophisticated program with a coach such as cogmed.com. If you have the time and resources, and you can find someone well trained in neurofeedback for TBI close to you (www.Bcia.org is an excellent resource), then meet with that person and start improving your brain function.

Brain exercise is one of the most challenging and empowering ways of recovery, like rehab for your brain. But it's only one part of the puzzle, so let's check out the next step to add to your program in my next chapter, which is getting a good night's rest.

Notes

1. Newberg A et al., Cerebral blood flow during meditative prayer: Preliminary findings and methodological issues, *Perceptual and Motor Skills* 97(2) (Oct 2003):145–50.

2. Davidson RJ, Kabat-Zinn J, Schumacher J et al. Alterations in brain and immune function produced by mindfulness meditation. *Psycho Med.* 2003;65(4):564–70.

3. Johansson B, Bjuhr H, Rönnbäck L. Mindfulness-based stress reduction (MBSR) improves long-term mental fatigue after stroke or traumatic brain injury. *Brain Inj.* 2012;26(13–14):1621–28. doi: 10.3109/02699052.2012.700082.

4. Bédard M, Mazmanian D, Felteau M et al. Pilot evaluation of a mindfulness-based intervention to improve quality of life among individuals who sustained traumatic brain injuries. *Dis Rehab.* 2003;25(13):722–31.

5. brainworksneurotherapy.com/history-and-development.

6. Duric NS, Assmus J, Gundersen DI et al. Neurofeedback for the treatment of children and adolescents with ADHD: a randomized and controlled clinical trial using parental reports. *BMC Psych.* 2012;12:107.

7. Monastra, VJ, Monastra DM, George S. The effects of stimulant therapy, EEG biofeedback, and parenting style on the primary symptoms of attention deficit/hyperactivity disorder. *Appl Psycho Biofeed.* 2002;27:237–41.

8. Casanova MF, El-Baz AS, Suri J, eds. *Imaging the brain in autism.* New York, NY: Springer; 2013.

9. May G, Benson R, Balon R et al. Neurofeedback and traumatic brain injury: a literature review. *Ann Clin Psych.* 2013;25(4):289–96.

10. Mather M. The emotion paradox in the aging brain. *Ann N Y Acad Sci.* 2012;1251(1):33–49.

11. Steiner NJ, Frenette EC, Rene KM et al. In-school neurofeedback training for ADHD: sustained improvements from a randomized control trial. *Pediatrics.* 2014:133(3).

10

SLEEP AND TRAUMATIC BRAIN INJURY

· ·

BRIGHT MINDS Principle

Sleep: Sleep is key for healing from brain injury and for having optimal brain function in general.

· ·

One time, I was giving a talk at a brain injury conference when an audience member asked an excellent question: "What causes sleep disruption after a TBI?"

"You know, I'm not sure what the mechanism is," I had to admit, even though many brain-injured patients report sleep problems and daytime fatigue. "I'll have to get back to you on that," I added, making a mental note to do some research and find out more information.

I knew that many patients, after a brain injury, often feel tired during the day and have trouble falling asleep at night. In those situations, the symptoms mimic regular forms of insomnia, but I also knew it was important to distinguish common sleep problems from brain injury–related sleep disruption.

Insomnia, which is widespread in our culture, is commonly caused by depression, anxiety, and stress. Other issues include, but are not limited to, emotional trauma, sleep apnea, chronic pain, bipolar disorder, worry, anger, and grief. After a TBI incident, typical sleep problems mean waking up throughout the night, not sleeping long enough, not getting enough deep sleep, and not getting enough REM sleep.[1] According to the National Institutes of Health, 30 percent to 70 percent of TBI patients have sleep problems. In my experience, I believe the percentage is closer to the upper number.[2]

Research has not fully uncovered exactly why this is the case, but the problem is likely due to disrupted neuronal cell firing. In other words, brain trauma can damage neurons to the point where they no longer fire properly or transition into rest mode when they should.

I would compare any TBI-related sleep problem to an annoying neighbor who keeps his music on just loud enough to keep you awake at night, but low enough during the day so that you can't hear what song is being played. In a similar way, injured brain cells are not going into "rest" mode at night or functioning well during the day. It's a lose-lose situation for patients who can't get the much-needed rest that's vital for healing.

One of the things a TBI sufferer needs the most is—you guessed it—consistent, healthy sleep. The fact that the damaged neurons cause sleep to be chronically disrupted makes it almost impossible to fully heal after a brain injury. This last statement is worth repeating and why this part of any brain-healing program is so important: *It is almost impossible to fully heal from a brain injury if sleep is chronically disrupted.*

This is why I've long believed that the lack of proper rest is a devastating problem.

But what happens to the brain when a TBI sufferer does not get sufficient sleep? As I discussed in chapter 4, the hormone chapter, part of the mechanism for healing is for the body to have sufficient growth hormone. Growth hormone is released during the deepest stages of sleep and is critical for healing an injured brain. If an injured brain keeps waking up every few hours, however, or does not get into deep stages of sleep, then insufficient growth hormone is released. When the cycle continues, your ability to function takes a nosedive.

On the other hand, some individuals sleep *too much* after a brain injury.[3] This is because the quality of their sleep is neither sufficiently deep nor restful, so they stay in bed until noon or later, fruitlessly trying to get the rest they need. Excess sleeping can actually make you more tired, especially when the sleep is of poor quality. When it comes to sleep, quality as well as quantity is important.

Another theory why people with TBI sleep too much is that part of the brain is damaged and is preventing the release of hypocretin, a wake-promoting chemical in the brain. Even six months after a head injury, 19 percent of patients still suffer from low hypocretin production. Maybe this is a survival mechanism to help TBI patients sleep longer when their brains need extra time to heal from trauma.[4,5]

Either way, under- or oversleeping can result in daytime

fatigue and cognitive problems such as difficulty concentrating and making good decisions.

Low levels of melatonin, a hormone secreted in the brain, may be keeping TBI patients from sleeping well. These secretions are based on circadian rhythms (the biological clock or rhythm that tells us when to wake and sleep) and in response to low light or darkness. When melatonin levels are normal, people become very sleepy at the end of a long day. When melatonin levels are not normal, people aren't sleepy and dread going to bed.

Does simply taking a melatonin supplement help with TBI-related sleep disruptions? One study showed that it does, and common sense says that it should. According to studies, melatonin improved sleep more than taking amitriptyline, a tricyclic antidepressant medication commonly prescribed for sleep disruptions, presumably by improving sleep quality in a group of TBI patients.[6] Giving patients melatonin versus amitriptyline also improved daytime alertness.

The other type of sleep disruption that may accompany TBI is sleep apnea, which is when you stop breathing while sleeping. If you have sleep apnea, you aren't getting enough oxygen to your brain while sleeping. The brain turns on the alarm bells, but this doesn't usually wake you to the point of consciousness; it does, however, disrupt how much deep sleep and REM sleep you get.

Sleep apnea is quite common in the general population as well as among TBI patients. From brain SPECT imaging, we can see decreased activity in a part of the brain called the parietal lobe, which is associated with obstructive sleep apnea.

Keep in mind that when you're sleeping, the brain goes through several stages of sleep. It's during the deepest stages of slumber that growth hormone is released, which is critical for healing.

Again, you could compare obstructive sleep apnea to music played by your neighbor: loud enough to keep you from much-needed deep sleep but not loud enough to wake you.

Dispelling a Sleep Myth

It's worth taking a moment to dispel a myth about sleep and its effects right after a brain injury.

For quite some time, it was believed that sleeping after a concussion or some type of significant brain injury could lead to more serious injury—or even death—if the person was not awakened every few hours. This idea may have come from a specific case study in which those with serious brain injuries had lost consciousness and then woken up. They were talking normally and all seemed fine, but they had bleeding inside their brains. Instead of receiving the appropriate medical care, they were allowed to fall back asleep. Sadly, and subsequently, they died.

While horrible for the families left behind, the good news is that these serious outcomes are quite rare when it comes to TBIs. Modern medical technology and awareness make it much easier to spot internal bleeding in the brain. If there is any suspicion that there may be bleeding in the brain, which can include such symptoms as dilated pupils and confusion, you should seek immediate medical help to receive a CT scan or MRI.

Today, for a minor hit to the head where the pupils are not dilated and there is no confusion, sleep is considered one of the best treatments. Most of the research now supports the idea that the brain needs to rest in order to heal, and that sleep is a natural mechanism to do so. Even more, keeping a person up and awake can actually interfere with the healing process. That's why it's important for you to sleep, and sleep well, right after a TBI or concussion because the brain needs rest.

Getting a Good Night's Sleep

Now that I've explored all the ways a TBI can disrupt your sleep and either impede or help your recovery, let's take a look at ways to improve your sleep patterns. The good news is that there's plenty of hope.

I'm sure you've seen the ads for prescription medications like Ambien, Lunesta, and Trazodone, among others. Are these the best route to take for insomnia? In my opinion, I would not advise you to take sleep medications like Ambien or benzodiazepines like temazepam, clonazepam, or Xanax. While these may help an individual fall asleep, there are considerable side effects and thery are not recommended for long-term use. Ask any flight attendant about Ambien, and they'll tell you horror stories about passengers who did bizarre things—"zombies," they call them—like taking off all their clothes and rushing into the first-class cabin after taking this commonly used sleep aid. Even for those who don't strip down in the economy section, such medications can cause problems with cognitive function, memory issue, and interference with sleep cycles. The reality is that prescription sleep medications don't give you a good quality of sleep and can cause memory problems.

With all these warnings in mind, I understand the strong pull to take *something* when you are desperate for sleep. Sometimes taking sleep medications in the short term is needed because not sleeping well can also have serious effects on memory, cognitive function, and your mood. In extreme cases, swallowing an occasional prescribed sleep aid such as Trazodone or doxepin may be advised, but only do so under your doctor's orders. Your prescribing health professional needs to work closely with you in these matters, as these medications can be habit forming.

Also, I've had many TBI patients who thought their memory problems were due to depression or early-onset dementia. In fact, however, their problems were due—at least in part—to the use of Ambien or clonazepam to help them sleep.

A patient named Julie had been worrying about memory problems that had started sometime in the past year. When I questioned her for details, she said her memory problems had actually started six months earlier. When I asked about her use of prescription medicine, she mentioned that she was taking clonazepam, a prescription drug used to treat anxiety attacks and insomnia. I knew that could be the issue. When I got her to taper off the clonazepam, her memory problems disappeared.

Note: It's important to work with your doctor before you change or stop these medications. If you have been taking one regularly and stop suddenly, that decision could have dangerous consequences. For example, abrupt cessation of benzodiazepines (e.g., clonazepam, Xanax, Halcion) has been known to cause seizures and rebound insomnia.

Natural Treatments for Insomnia: Sleep Hygiene

When it comes to getting good sleep, you have to start with your bedroom, which should be reserved for sleep and sex only.

Make sure your room is very dark and quiet; even the red numerals of a digital clock can hinder your ability to fall asleep. The amount of darkness in the bedroom is important; in one study, patients with TBI had much lower levels of melatonin secretion even in low-light conditions.[7] If your room is not entirely dark or quiet, wear an eye mask and earplugs to help you fall into a deeper sleep. This is especially helpful if you happen to share your bed with your spouse or partner or with a dog or a cat.

Go to bed around the same time each night, typically when you start to feel sleepy. This may be much sooner than you realize. For most people, the time is around 9 to 10 p.m. While it may seem obvious, feeling drowsy is a great signal that your body is ready for bed.

If you ignore your body's signals and decide to stay up, you may encounter the "second wind" phenomenon that many of us experience. When you keep going at night—working on a project, socializing with friends, dancing in a loud disco—the body releases cortisol, a stress hormone, which all but guarantees to keep you awake. When you do finally go to bed, perhaps after midnight or later, you will still have all that extra cortisol circulating through your bloodstream, which will make it much harder to fall asleep and stay asleep. Your odds of experiencing a truly restful sleep are greatly diminished.

Getting exercise during the day is another way to help ensure a good night's sleep. Don't go to the gym after dinner, however. Many people need a time buffer between exercise and sleep because exercise is so energizing. If you do exercise after 6 p.m., make sure you finish at least two hours before bedtime.

I will say, though, that I've known individuals who actually sleep better after exercising and burning off stress from the day, and that includes myself. Sometimes I'll take a fifteen-minute easy jog after the kids go to bed at 8 p.m., and I sleep much better at 10 or 10:30. If the *only* time you can exercise is after the workday or dinner, then see how you sleep after each session of vigorous exercise.

You will have to be smart about what you're doing and consuming in the last few hours of the day and your bedroom environment. In this day and age, we tend to keep our screens on until late into the evening, either watching TV, working on the computer, or scrolling through social media on our smartphones. The blue light emitted from these devices is known to suppress the release of melatonin, which can negatively affect both your ability to fall asleep and the quality and depth of your sleep.[8] Even having your phone in the bedroom can cause sleep disruption, regardless if you turn off the sound. You'll still hear the smartphone buzzing when a text, email, Instagram, or WhatsApp message comes through.

It's best to turn the damn thing off and leave it in the kitchen, where it can be charging. If you leave your smartphone on your nightstand, your subconscious mind will know it's there and will be working overtime wondering what notifications and messages you could be getting. Studies even show that a wooden "phone"—an object that represents a phone—can be distracting because of our association with the shape and feel of a telephone handset. If you've been using your smartphone as an alarm clock, which means you *have* to leave it on, that's no excuse. You can get a good old-fashioned and silent alarm clock for just a few bucks these days.

If you have to have screen time at night, one strategy is to wear glasses with amber lenses when looking at your screen. The amber lenses block the blue wavelength of light, causing the body to think it's dark outside. Blue wavelength of light is the most potent form of circadian rhythm signaling, and therefore the most important you want to block out.[9]

When I really want to get a deep sleep, I wear an eye mask and earplugs—not because my wife snores (she doesn't), but because I'm a light sleeper. When I block out sound and light this way, I sink down into even-deeper sleep than on nights that I don't.

One dilemma faced by many of my patients is a loud sleep partner. If your partner snores like a chugging locomotive or has sleep apnea, all that noise can disrupt your ability to get a good night's sleep. I don't normally advocate sleeping in separate bedrooms, but sometimes that's necessary—especially if the other person is unwilling to get assessed and treated for snoring or sleep apnea.

Sleeping in the same bed or same room with someone can make it more difficult to stay asleep. Even if your co-sleeper isn't a snorer, maybe he or she is disruptive in other ways. Your partner could be a classic sleepwalker, someone who talks or mumbles out loud in their sleep, a cover stealer, or someone who is restless and flip-flops constantly throughout the night. In those cases, wearing sensory-dulling devises like earplugs and an eye mask will help drown out your co-sleeper's nocturnal movements and sounds.

Melatonin

As I mentioned before, melatonin can serve as a great, natural alternative to prescription sleep aids and is the sleep aid that most people tell me they've already tried when I ask them what they have used for sleeping. But it doesn't work for everybody. In those cases, I will ask my patients to explain why melatonin did nothing for them. Perhaps melatonin didn't work because the dosage was either too low, too high, or the timing of when they took it was the problem. I tell patients that melatonin can be a finicky supplement for some people.

The good news is that melatonin is exceedingly safe. You may not be aware that melatonin is given frequently to cancer patients—up to 20 mg—for its antioxidant benefit alone.[10]

I don't recommend taking that much, especially if you're trying to fall asleep. Since the body produces about 0.5 mg of melatonin at night while sleeping, I recommend starting with that amount. Another strategy is to take this dose at dusk and right before bedtime. Be sure to wear your blue-blocker glasses during the hours before you lay your head on the pillow, but that's only if you're *really* having trouble falling asleep.

The idea is to reset normal circadian rhythms. What is

probably most helpful is to get into a sleep routine as noted above, going to bed at approximately the same time every night, and getting yourself ready for sleep by doing relaxing things—and definitely not raising your blood pressure by watching political news and commentary shows on TV.

If the lower dose of melatonin doesn't work after a couple nights, then try a higher dose. You can safely try 1–3 mg to start, then adjusting the dose up gradually every few nights until you find the right sweet spot.

But know this: if there is no effect at 10 mg, then melatonin is not going to help.

That said, I've been a melatonin fan for a long time. When I worked in a treatment center, I remember one young man who was struggling with severe depression and drug addiction. An attending physician prescribed 200 mg of Seroquel, a powerful antipsychotic medication, to help him sleep. Even with that heavy dose, he was still waking up in the night with insomnia. He was then given 3 mg of melatonin as a sample, and he came back the next day asking, "What was that stuff you gave me? It knocked me out." Needless to say, he requested melatonin from then on.

Another strategy is to combine both an immediate and controlled-release melatonin that can work together as a "one-two punch," so to speak. Melatonin has a half-life of around four hours, so while it's instrumental in helping you get to sleep, it doesn't necessarily help you *stay* asleep. By taking a second, controlled-release dose of melatonin, you can prevent waking up in the middle of the night or early morning. I've found that this approach works especially well with TBI patients.[11]

Even if you aren't having sleep problems, melatonin has neuroprotective and antioxidant effects, so taking it after a TBI is always going to be helpful.[12]

Magnesium

Magnesium is a mineral found in green leafy vegetables, and because many of us don't eat as much salad as we should, we don't get enough magnesium in the body. In fact, 60 percent of Americans are deficient in this vital nutrient that regulates muscle and nerve function, blood sugar levels, and blood pressure and helps make protein, bone, and DNA within the body.[13] While calcium helps muscles to contract, magnesium helps them to relax.

I often recommend a magnesium supplement to help my patients sleep. Normally 250–500 mg is all it takes. Some types of magnesium, such as magnesium oxide or magnesium citrate, in higher doses will cause loose stools if taken all at once. These types aren't as well absorbed into the bloodstream and end up staying in the gut, pulling water toward them, which loosens the stool. These forms of magnesium are well tolerated, however, if taken in smaller doses and increased gradually over a couple of days.

Other forms of magnesium, such as magnesium glycinate and magnesium threonate, are more highly absorbed, so lower doses are sufficient. Magnesium glycinate (250–500 mg) and magnesium threonate (155 mg) taken at bedtime are superb natural muscle and mind relaxants.

211

Tryptophan

Tryptophan, an amino acid, is highly sedating and sleep-promoting. It also is a precursor to serotonin, which means this essential nutrient can help with depressive symptoms. One caution, though: if you are taking an antidepressant such as a selective serotonin reuptake inhibitor (SSRI) (e.g., Prozac, Zoloft, or Paxil), which also affects the serotonin pathways, please check with your doctor before trying tryptophan for insomnia. The risk is a potentially life-threatening condition called serotonin syndrome.

Tryptophan (1,000–2,000 mg) before bedtime will help you fall asleep and stay asleep and may also improve mood. Or you can eat foods high in tryptophan such as turkey, cheese, yogurt, fish, and eggs. Remember, the body can't make tryptophan, so diet or supplements must supply this essential amino acid that's important for so many bodily functions.

Passionflower Extract

Passionflower extract is an herbal anxiolytic, meaning it "cuts through" anxiety. In several studies, this extract has been compared to benzodiazepines—similar in effect but without the cognitive dulling side effects.[14]

Phosphatidyl Serine (PS)

Phosphatidyl serine is a membrane phospholipid, meaning it actually forms the cell membrane that makes up all our cells.

Ten percent of our brain is made of phosphatidyl serine and is used for several reasons in regard to sleep:

- It helps by blunting the effect of cortisol, especially at higher doses (300–600 mg).[15]

- Studies reveal that it helps with memory concerns and concentration, such as in ADHD.[16]

Do You Really Need Eight Straight Hours of Sleep?

I heard an interesting historical review of sleep on public radio recently. Two hundred years ago, before the invention of the electric light bulb, people tended to go to sleep soon after it became dark—7 p.m. or even earlier most of the year, because Daylight Savings Time hadn't been implemented yet. They would then sleep for four hours or so, and then wake up for an hour or two to do some more work, knit a sweater, play card games, or get a small bite to eat. Then they would fall back to sleep for another four hours and awaken at daybreak to start their morning chores.

I tend to believe that good sleep does not have to involve sleeping eight hours in a row. As a matter of fact, this type of sleep pattern is a fairly modern phenomenon. The important thing is to get enough deep sleep, wherein REM stage is reached. (It's common knowledge that it takes the average person about one and a half to two hours to reach the REM stage.)

If you wake up in the middle of the night and can't get back to sleep right away, don't be overly alarmed. Simply use the time to relax, think, read, pray, or even talk with your spouse—if he or she is awake, of course! If you cannot fall back asleep for the rest of the night, though, see your doctor.

I used to think that "the perfect night's rest" had to consist of a single, undisturbed block of eight hours of sleep. However, in my practice, I've found this kind of mind-set can actually cause worsening sleep problems because of the anxiety and stress and pressure that we put on ourselves. In that sense, I think we are too rigid with our ideas of what sleep—great sleep—should be.

The main goal is to get the sleep *you* need—especially if you are recovering from a TBI. Your body is a sensitive instrument, and if you are not getting the sleep you need, your body will let you know.

To that point, my sincere hope is that these sleep recommendations will help you get the quality rest you need for your injured brain.

After all, sleep is critical. For without sleep, how can the brain heal?

Notes

1. Grima N, Ponsford J, Rajaratnam SM et al. Sleep disturbances in traumatic brain injury: a meta-analysis. *J Clin Sleep Med.* 2016;12(3):419–28.

2. Vioila-Saltzman M, Watson N. Traumatic brain injury and sleep disorders. *Neurol Clin.* 2012;30(4):1299–1312.

3. Kempf J, Kaiser P, Werth E et al. Sleep-wake disturbances 3 years after traumatic brain injury. *J Neurol Neurosurg Psych.* 2010;81(12):1402–5. doi:10.1136/jnnp.2009.201913.

4. Baumann CR, Werth E, Stocker R et al. Sleep–wake disturbances 6 months after traumatic brain injury: a prospective study. *Brain.* 2007;130(7):1873–83.

5. Orff HJ, Ayalon L, Drummond SP. Traumatic brain injury and sleep disturbance: a review of current research. *J Head Trauma Rehab.* 2009;24(3):155–65.

6. Kemp S, Biswas R, Neumann V et al. The value of melatonin for sleep disorders occurring post-head injury: a pilot RCT. *Brain Inj.* 2004;18(9):911–19.

7. Shekleton JA, Parcell DL, Redman JR et al. Sleep disturbance and melatonin levels following traumatic brain injury. *Neurology.* 2010;74(21):1732–38.

8. Cajochen C, Münch M, Kobialka S et al. High sensitivity of human melatonin, alertness, thermoregulation, and heart rate to short wavelength light. *J Clin Endocrinol Metab.* 2005;90(3):1311–16.

9. Burkhart K, Phelps JR. Amber lenses to block blue light and improve sleep: a randomized trial. *Chronobiol Int.* 2009;26(8):1602–12. doi: 10.3109/07420520903523719.

10. Ya L, Sha L, Yue Z et al. Melatonin for the prevention and treatment of cancer. *Oncotarget.* 2017;8(24):39896–921.

11. Grima NA, Rajaratnam SMW, Mansfield D et al. Efficacy of melatonin for sleep disturbance following traumatic brain injury: a randomised controlled trial. *BMC Med.* 2018;16:8.

12. Osier N, McGreevy E, Pham L et al. Melatonin as a therapy for traumatic brain injury: a review of published evidence. *Int J Mol Sci.* 2018;19(5):1539.

13. King D, Mainous A, Geesey M et al. Dietary magnesium and C-RP levels. *J Am College of Nutrition.* 2005;24(3):166–71.

14. Akhondzadeh S, Naghavi HR, Vazirian M et al. Passionflower in the treatment of generalized anxiety: a pilot double blind randomized controlled trial with oxazepam. *J Clin Pharm Ther.* 2001;26(5):363–67.

15. Starks MA, Starks SL, Kingsley M et al. The effects of phosphatidylserine on endocrine response to moderate intensity exercise. *J Inter Soc Sports Nutr.* 2008;5(11).

16. Hirayama S, Terasawa K, Rabeler R et al. The effect of phosphatidyl serine administration on memory and symptoms of attention deficit hyperactivity disorder: a randomized, double blind, placebo controlled clinical trial. *J Huan Nutr Diet.* 2014;27(Suppl 2):284–91.

11

EXERCISE AND TRAUMATIC BRAIN INJURY

BRIGHT MINDS Principles

Blood flow: One of the best ways to increase blood flow to the brain is through exercise, especially aerobic exercise.

Mental health: The effects of aerobic exercise on mood are well known and this becomes even more important when you have an injured brain.

Immunity: Aerobic exercise is one of the best ways to help support immune system function.

Diabesity: Regular aerobic exercise will help drive down blood sugar and prevent insulin resistance. The brain, which is starving for nutrition after a brain injury, needs exercise in order to have optimal blood glucose control.

••

We are made to move!

Throughout most of human evolutionary history, we have taken part in high amounts of physical activity. Think about the migration of mankind from Asia, across the land bridge that once connected that continent to North America (or what is known today as the Bering Strait). During the last Ice Age, between 15,000 and 30,000 years ago, nomads from Asia walked thousands of miles over many generations to reach North America, Central America, and South America. That's thousands of miles on foot, living off the land for sustenance. It seems absolutely incredible today!

Let's move forward in time to more civilized and complex societies such as the ancient Romans. When Julius Caesar conducted his campaign to conquer the Gauls (in modern-day France), his legionnaires walked more than twenty miles per day in hobnailed leather sandals. Over the course of one four-year military campaign, Caesar's legions marched thousands of miles, building timber-walled encampments at the end of each day, and fighting major battles throughout their military campaign. Talk about being in good shape!

As a species that has been evolving for 100,000–200,000 years, hunting and gathering simply became a part of life, causing entire cultures to stay on the move. In his book *Go Wild* about exercise and the brain, psychiatrist Dr. John Ratey describes the process of moving from a hunting and gathering culture to a more agrarian, less-mobile one. He said that as societies began to settle in one place, the human brain had to figure out what to do after hunting and killing animals, and how to store the berries and nuts that had been gathered.

There is a link, then, between movement and brain activity. In modern societies—especially in more affluent cities and nations where more jobs are more sedentary—exercise is no longer a natural, normal part of daily life. In other words, most people living in First World nations do not exercise or even walk much to survive. Instead, many of us sit for long stretches of time—in our cars during long commutes or on the bus or train to work, and then we sit in an office chair in our cubicles all day long.

So what effect does this less-physical lifestyle have on our brains? A lot, because just as exercise enhances memory and thinking skills, a lack of exercise worsens overall brain function.

When studying the brain and its relationship to exercise, I need to talk about a protein called BDNF, or brain-derived neurotrophic factor. BDNF increases the sprouting of new neurons as well as the growth and increase in connections of existing neurons. BDNF also protects the brain.

Research clearly shows that BDNF is increased by exercise more than by any other factor. Other things that increase BDNF include antidepressants, niacin, and the essential fatty acid DHA. But of all these factors, exercise is by far the most potent and effective step for increasing BDNF.

So what is incredibly helpful after a brain injury? What increases the budding, sprouting, and growth of new neurons? The answer is BDNF!

But BDNF is not the only reason to start exercising after a TBI. We know that exercise improves mood, cardiovascular fitness, and even self-esteem,[1] and oftentimes after a TBI or concussion, it's common to have some level of depression or loss of identity. Think of the college athlete who is not allowed to play after making it all the way to the collegiate level to play Division I soccer.

Which leads me to an important question: When is it safe to start exercising after a traumatic or chronic brain injury? As discussed in chapter 6 regarding different nutrients for a TBI, some caution needs to be exercised (no pun intended) when starting back into a vigorous exercise routine. If you start exercising too soon after an acute brain injury, you can actually worsen the healing process.

Though there is scant research on this subject, one study has shown interesting results. Mice were given a brain injury and then assessed a week later. During those seven days, they had access to an exercise wheel in their cage. At the one-week mark following an acute TBI, they showed less neuroplasticity and less BDNF. In other words, rather than accelerating their TBI recovery, exercise seemed to impede it.

But when the mice were only allowed to exercise at five weeks post-injury, they experienced improved memory and decreased the size of the brain lesion from the injury.[2] So timing is everything. Exercising too soon after an injury can slow recovery, whereas exercise several weeks later can make all the difference. These types of studies have been repeated in humans, but I must caution you that there is still much debate about when and how to return to exercise after a brain injury.

Coaches and athletes know that returning to a sport too soon after injury is going to worsen recovery, yet exercise is sometimes one of the best things you can do for a TBI. So what's the right answer? When should one start exercising after a concussion or TBI?

A rule of thumb, especially if you are five weeks post-injury or later, is to exercise up to the point where you start having worsening symptoms. Then you have to back off. For instance, if a fifteen-minute intense run causes you to have headaches afterward, but a ten-minute jog leaves you feeling great, then stick to ten minutes even though you may have the energy to do another five or ten minutes of running.

The type of exercise is important too. Sometimes running on pavement or concrete can be too jarring, especially for those with sensitive injuries, so dust off that bicycle or use an elliptical machine or StairMaster in the gym. Swimming laps is also a great way to exercise because of its low-impact overall body workout.

Jane loved her weekly aerobics classes at the gym, but after her car accident, she wasn't able to continue this for several weeks without getting a headache and feeling dizzy afterward. She had to wait four weeks before she could even start taking long walks again. Once she did resume exercising, her recovery sped up, and she was able to add a few minutes to her walks each week, eventually getting to the point where she could go back to her aerobics class. Initially, she was only able to complete half of her workout class, but in time she was able to get back to her regular routine.

A return to vigorous physical activity must be done with caution and depends upon the severity of the injury. Keep in mind that most of the benefits that I describe in this chapter are meant for TBI patients whose injuries are three months old or more.

Based on research, we have learned that strength training, including weight lifting and resistance exercise, does not have a big effect on BDNF. I love resistance training and think it's an important way to increase other factors that help with healing, but resistance training or strength training is not nearly as effective for TBI recovery as cardiovascular exercise.

A 2013 study demonstrated that any type of exercise that gets the heart pumping will produce BDNF. That said, the study did demonstrate that the more intense the exercise, the more BDNF is produced. Results revealed that doing cardio for forty minutes (at 80 percent of maximum heart rate) was more effective at producing the most BDNF than doing twenty minutes of similar exercise.[3]

In other words, the more intense and the longer the duration of the cardiovascular exercise, the more BDNF is released.

Another benefit of exercise as it relates to brain healing is an increase in human growth hormone. As I discussed in chapter 4, human growth hormone is commonly found to be low after brain injury due to a damaged pituitary gland. Human growth hormone helps with growth and healing from TBI and can be increased with exercise in both young and older adults.[4,5]

As a matter of fact, human growth hormone can be increased dramatically by doing special types of exercise such as interval training. Interval training, which means going fast or running fast out of the gate—also known as "bursting"—and then going slower, is perhaps the most efficient way to increase human growth hormone.

Why does bursting-type exercise increase human growth hormone? We have three types of muscle fibers: slow, fast, and superfast. The superfast muscle fibers are the only ones that—when triggered—produce human growth hormone.

What works these superfast fibers the most? You guessed it . . . going all out or as fast as you can, using the maximum effort possible. It's estimated that after a session of interval training, the human growth hormone goes up by 500 percent for the next two hours.

To make the most of this growth hormone–releasing effect, it's best to avoid sugary foods and drinks after you finish exercising. The reason for this is because when sweets or carbs are consumed, insulin is released, which causes reabsorption of human growth hormone.

Avoiding sugar and carbs after exercise is the opposite of what is typically discussed for post-exercise recovery. When I was playing soccer and running in my glory days, I was trained to consume carbs and sugars before, during, and after training and competition to speed up recovery. This strategy was designed originally for elite athletes who need to bounce back quickly—and must consume a lot of calories right away. Eating carbs helps them recover faster but that doesn't help boost human growth hormone levels. Actually, an influx of carbs will drop your growth hormone, so don't load up on sugary sweets after intense exercise. Now that I am an "older" athlete, I don't pound Gatorade after a hard run because I don't want to flush away the hard-earned human growth hormone that I produced. I wait about thirty minutes, and then I have a protein shake or a high-protein, higher-in-fat meal. In addition, after age thirty, your levels of human growth hormone start to decline, so adopting "bursting" exercise will help keep your human growth hormone levels up.

Several years ago, the American College of Cardiology changed their guidelines for recommended exercise times and amounts. The old recommendation was that the average adult should participate in aerobic exercise for thirty minutes five times a week. The newer guidelines recommend interval training as the preferred aerobic exercise for twenty minutes five times a week.

When it comes to interval training, the importance is in the burst, where you alter your speed and intensity from low to high quickly. This type of exercise is particularly beneficial for your brain. This is how a typical interval training session might go:

- Warm up for ninety seconds at a slow pace
- Then "burst"—or go about 60–80 percent of your maximum effort for thirty seconds
- Then keep a moderate pace for ninety seconds
- Then "burst" again for thirty seconds
- Repeat until you have achieved eight bursts
- Cool down for ninety seconds or longer

From personal experience, I've found this type of burst exercise to be very difficult, and you'll likely have the same experience, especially if you aren't used to it. If you are going to run or sprint your intervals, make sure you first jog approximately half a mile at a slow pace, and then stretch out. Properly warming up and stretching your muscles will greatly reduce the chances of your pulling a muscle. Also, sprinting does increase your risk of pulling a muscle or injuring tender joints and tendons. Some of my patients do this type of interval training at a local track, preferably synthetic, as it's gentler on the joints. Wherever you choose to run, avoid running on hard surfaces such as pavement and concrete, as they can be very hard on your joints and skeletal system.

Interval training can be done with any form of exercise, including running, elliptical, rowing machine, StairMaster, swimming, biking, recumbent exercise bike, upright stationary bike, and even walking. One of my favorite ways to get a burst workout in the gym is pedaling a recumbent bike.

The important thing is to alternate between going faster and then slower. The reason this works is because the body likes to adapt. If you keep changing things up, the body doesn't get a chance to adapt and therefore must compensate and grow much stronger in the process. This is why the American Heart Association recommends interval training after heart surgery to help speed recovery.

When I'm not in the gym, my exercise of choice is running. Jogging is not for everyone, but for me, as a busy doctor and dad of three young kids, it's ideal. Running is simple and time efficient, as I can get a great workout in less than a half hour.

Then again, you have to like running. I'm grateful that I was first introduced to running by my fourth-grade teacher, Mrs. Beckham, who had a great sense of humor and was sharp as a tack, even though she was probably in her late sixties when she taught me.

Mrs. Beckham loved to run and bicycle. She read us the story of Glenn Cunningham, a Kansas native whose legs were badly burned in a fire in the one-room schoolhouse when he was eight years old. Doctors recommended amputation, but Glenn fought to keep his leg. Even though he was unable to walk for two years, with great determination he started walking and then running again. Seventeen years later, Cunningham held the world record for the mile in 1934.

I was inspired by his story and by Mrs. Beckham, who preached the value of running and determination and told us that we could all become good runners. The entire fourth-grade class entered the annual two-mile Wichita River Run and got a local running club to sponsor us with brand-new running shoes. I was thrilled to be a part of such an event, and I've run ever since.

I'll grant you that running is certainly not for everyone. My wife, Drie, prefers doing long vigorous walks or the elliptical or treadmill at the gym, and I can't blame her, since it's often rainy and cold in Seattle. But gyms cost money or can be inconvenient or too distant. If that's your case, you can leave your home and run around the neighborhood to get a good workout in a hurry—and all it costs is a decent pair of running shoes.

Here are some other ideas to get a good workout quickly and efficiently:

- Jumping rope
- Running in place
- Doing calisthenics such as push-ups, sit-ups, or burpees, which is a push-up followed by standing up and jumping in the air with your hands over your head

You can find a lot of great workouts on the Web, including videos on YouTube. Wherever you work out and however you do it, the important thing is to get your heart rate up and start pumping out some BDNF and human growth hormone.

The website mybrainfitlife.com is a great resource for workouts. Not only does the portal provide a like-minded support community, but the website has features that allow you to track your progress. An added bonus is access to online coaches who can help you if you need it.

Planning your exercise routine and finding support are probably the most critical aspects to integrating exercise into your life. Keep these things in mind:

1. Frequency. How many times a week do you plan to start exercising now versus your goal that you want to work up to in the future? **Note:** it's much better to set a modest goal and surpass it than it is to start too high and not meet it. If you are currently not working out at all, a good starting point might be to exercise two or three times a week and then work up from there.

2. Duration. Plan on starting with less time versus more time. If doing intervals, consider starting with two or three "bursts" and then working up to eight or so. The goal should be to leave the workout with some energy left over and a feeling that you could do another interval if you wanted to. That way you won't be dead tired and have a negative association with the workout.

3. Support. Is there anyone who you can work out with or meet at a gym or in the neighborhood for a walk? Even the family dog can help you get outdoors and moving around.

4. Find a good gym. These days gym memberships can be quite reasonable, especially if you shop for a deal. While a fancy gym with all sorts of amenities is nice, a "no frills" place or a local YMCA may be all you need.

The benefit of a gym is that you can find community as well as exercise classes. The nice thing about exercise classes is that they are activities that happen at a scheduled time, so you can plan around them. Classes offer more accountability, particularly if they are on your calendar. Your mind-set will change from "Do I feel like going?" to "I have to get to my class."

I've always been a runner, so I never thought I would go to an exercise or aerobics class—or be happy exercising this way. But after trying a few of them—and there were times when I was the only guy in the class—I found myself trying things I had never done before. I was also introduced to important exercises that I was missing when working out on my own, such as exercises that strengthened my core and upper body. When I started adding one workout class per week to my running schedule, my fitness improved and working out became more enjoyable. The extra work on my core and upper body helped with tension in my neck and back.

When it comes to exercise, remember that you're not required to walk twenty-plus miles per day in leather sandals and a tunic like a Roman legionnaire. But you have to get up and move, which isn't easy in the sedentary culture we live in. But more than just getting the right amount of aerobic exercise, you need to strengthen your back, neck, and abdomen. Any physical therapist or chiropractor will tell you that sitting for long stretches at a time—where you tend to strain forward to peer at computer screens—can wreak havoc on your body.

The more sitting and driving you do, the more you need to exercise your upper body in the proper way. It's incredibly important to strengthen your core (stomach and lower back) and stretch the muscles in your back, legs, and hips. Focus on exercises that counteract your tendency to lean forward with your back and neck.

Exercise is one of those things in life—like eating healthy—that can be deceptively hard to do, especially consistently. If you're like me, the intentions are always there, but the tyranny of the urgent and the crazy pace of life can really sidetrack anyone. But remind yourself that the only person who is going to get you exercising on a regular schedule is . . . you!

So take advantage of every "help" you can, including finding a friend or buddy who will exercise with you. Look for online communities for your favorite sports or pastimes and get involved. Being around like-minded people will encourage and inspire you. For those suffering from TBI, the benefits are huge when you receive the "bonus benefits" of increased BDNF and human growth hormone.

Of all the things under your control as a TBI survivor, exercise can bring dramatic, nearly instant positive results in your journey toward healing.

You can do it. Surround yourself with a small team of cheerleaders that can help you along the way.

You won't regret it at all!

Notes

1. Schwandt M, Harris JE, Thomas S et al. Feasibility and effect of aerobic exercise for lowering depressive symptoms among individuals with traumatic brain injury: a pilot study. *J Head Trauma Rehab.* 2012;27(2):99–103.

2. Piao CS, Stoica BA, Wu J et al. Late exercise reduces neuroinflammation and cognitive dysfunction after traumatic brain injury. *Neurobiol Dis.* 2013;54:252–63.

3. Schmolesky MT, Webb DL, Hansen RA. The effects of aerobic exercise intensity and duration on levels of brain-derived neurotrophic factor in healthy men. *J Sports Sci Med.* 2013;12(3):502–11.

4. Kyun Jeon Y, Ho Ha C. Expression of brain-derived neurotrophic factor, IGF-1 and cortisol elicited by regular aerobic exercise in adolescents. *J Phys Ther Sci.* 2015;27(3):737–41.

5. Lanfranco F, Gianotti L, Giordano R. Ageing, growth hormone, and physical performance. *J Endocrinol Invest.* 2003;26(9):861–72.

12

HYPERBARIC OXYGEN FOR TRAUMATIC BRAIN INJURY

• •

BRIGHT MINDS Principles

Blood flow: Hyperbaric oxygen activates the brain and brings about increased blood flow to the entire brain.

Retirement/aging: As the brain ages you will have more difficulty healing from a brain injury. Hyperbaric oxygen speeds up the healing process.

Inflammation: Hyperbaric oxygen helps to lower brain and body inflammation levels and increase antioxidant defenses.

Head trauma: Hyperbaric oxygen is one of the most helpful treatments for helping to heal a brain injury.

Immunity/Infection: Hyperbaric oxygen supports the immune system and may directly help to eradicate certain types of infections such as Lyme disease.

Neurohormone deficiencies: Hyperbaric oxygen turns on growth factors, which helps to increase brain healing.

• •

One "magic bullet" does not exist for the treatment of TBI, but if I had to pick one therapy that has been shown to improve healing from brain injury rather consistently, then it would be hyperbaric oxygen therapy (HBOT). This is because it helps to address so many of the BRIGHT MINDS principles listed above.

What is HBOT? Therapy begins with using a hyperbaric chamber, which is a pressurized compartment with differing concentrations of oxygen. These chambers are commonly used for decompression from scuba diving–related accidents known as "the bends." The diver goes into the chamber, where he breathes 100 percent oxygen and the pressure is increased to drive out the nitrogen bubbles inside his body and replace those with oxygen.

These chambers are often used in hospitals for wounds that won't heal such as diabetic ulcers and strokes. The chambers are also used for the treatment of brain injuries at a lower pressure than would be used for scuba divers. I like the analogy of the nonhealing wound because that is really what many brain injuries are—and you just can't see them.

The risks are that because you're under pressure while in the chamber breathing as close to 100 percent oxygen as possible, your ears or lungs could be damaged, especially if you have sinus problems like a sinus infection. Oxygen poisoning and claustrophobia are other risks as well. Plus, treatments are time intensive and costly.

Most of the time, though, it's worth it. I love the story of Brett Baca, the son of Darren and Jill Baca, who used HBOT to heal after suffering a severe concussion while playing college football. Likely it was an effect of cumulative concussions, but Brett's last injury pushed him over the edge. He suffered migraine headaches, racing thoughts, brain fog, dizziness, and light sensitivity. He stayed in his dark dorm room 24/7 and became more irritable and depressed each day.

When Brett didn't get any better, his parents brought him home to San Francisco to try and find answers on their own. Eventually, they took him to the Amen Clinic in San Francisco to have him assessed using SPECT imaging. The scan showed years of injury to his brain from playing football and other sports. Brett started taking hyperbaric oxygen treatments, and after just ten sessions, he began to feel better. His stamina returned, his headaches lessened, and he was able to return to light exercise. With subsequent sessions in the chamber, he continued to feel improvements in energy and eventually made a complete recovery.

From my experience, a hyperbaric chamber does not deliver for every patient like it did for Brett Baca, but I've heard plenty of patients tell me, "This turned my life around" or "My brain fog lifted after the tenth session," so I think using a hyperbaric chamber is definitely worth considering. I think the key for HBOT is that it tends to help "boost" the healing process versus many other types of treatment.

The favorable results are often sustained if HBOT is done

along with a proper diet and exercise program, getting sufficient sleep, optimizing hormones, and using supplementation. If these foundational steps are not addressed, then even if improvements are made with HBOT, the improvements will not be sustained.

Mark Affleck was a CEO who thought he had escaped the effects of concussions he received while playing high school football. When he came in to see my colleague Dr. Amen, Mark was depressed, fatigued, dizzy, and under extreme stress. He had seen his primary care doctor as well as a neurologist, and they both attributed his symptoms to stress. They recommended that he rest more.

What was clear from SPECT imaging was that the combination of a weakened brain from previous injury and the stress of his present job was contributing to his symptoms. Dr. Amen immediately prescribed forty sessions of HBOT, and within the first five sessions, Mark began to feel his energy returning.

At the completion of forty sessions, he felt much better than before. His dizziness had ceased, his energy improved, and he felt enthusiasm for the first time in a long while. He had his SPECT scans repeated, and they showed significant improvement.

Several years later, however, some of the symptoms returned, such as a lowering mood and feeling fatigued. Dr. Amen wisely asked me to work him up for other contributing factors. His hormones were low, especially testosterone and thyroid. When we treated those, Mark had a return of energy and improved mood. He also did another round of forty hyperbaric chamber sessions. More than two years have passed since then, and today he's still doing well and has had no return of symptoms. *The key, I believe, was addressing both the underlying physical/metabolic issues and giving him a healing treatment such as HBOT.*

Taking Over

We see time and again that people can heal years after a TBI. So why is the brain able to heal after many years when most of the healing is thought to occur after a year and no further improvements can be expected after that?

One theory of why brains can heal after significant injury even years later is that the cells were just "dazed" and became "dormant." Even though it was thought that brain cells were killed by brain injury, they were actually in a "gray zone" where they were not fully functioning but alive. The cells are still alive, but because of their low activity, there is less blood supply, which makes them less active, so it's like they are on life support without fully recovering. The idea is that neuronal brain cells are in a state of a suspended animation, waiting to be resuscitated.

With an added infusion of nutrients, cellular energy, and oxygen, they *can* heal and recover. By supplying the cells with an enhanced oxygen-rich environment, the cells are able to become more metabolically active. These more active cells then recruit extra blood vessels to support their activity, and that's when new capillary formation happens. With new and more abundant blood supply, damaged cells can maintain their improved state.

What I have just described is the theory—which has not been definitively proven yet—of how HBOT works. One of HBOT's biggest proponents is Dr. Paul Harch, author of *The Oxygen Revolution*, who has hundreds of successful patient stories and has been working in this field and publishing key research for over thirty-five years.

Dr. Harch points out that after the brain cells have revved up and laid down new capillary beds, the increased activity of the cells should persist and sessions in the hyperbaric chamber may be stopped. So how long should HBOT take? From my experience, as well as a general consensus in the field, I would say that HBOT takes about eight weeks at a minimum and should be done sequentially. When using a hyperbaric oxygen chamber, this process takes a minimum of forty hours of sessions to help traumatic brain injury.

Stories of Healing

After hearing many stories of improvement, Xavier Figuero, a PhD researcher, decided to study the effect of HBOT on a young man who had suffered a catastrophic brain injury while playing football five years earlier. The story started right here in the state of Washington. Zackery Lystedt was a thirteen-year-old football player who took a serious hit during a game. After sitting out for fifteen minutes, he was put back in and caught a pass. While trying to score a touchdown, Zack was hit on the goal line—hard.

This time he had a massive brain bleed and collapsed on the field. After three months in and out of comas, and then over the next thirteen months, he relearned how to walk and talk, but Zack still has difficulty walking and talking, and because of his massive brain bleed, it's likely that he will never be the same again.

Because of Zack's life-changing injury, his family did not want another player to have to endure what they went through. They worked with Washington State lawmakers to pass the Zackery Lystedt Law to protect young athletes if they are suspected of having a concussion. The law, which has now been passed in all fifty states, says that the player must be evaluated by a healthcare professional trained in the evaluation of concussion prior to returning to play.

Zackery, as part of his therapy, underwent forty sessions of HBOT, and the before-and-after SPECT scans can be seen below. The results speak for themselves with the arrows showing the most improvement. The goal, of course, is not to expect reversal of his severe brain injury but to see what effect HBOT can have at improving brain function.

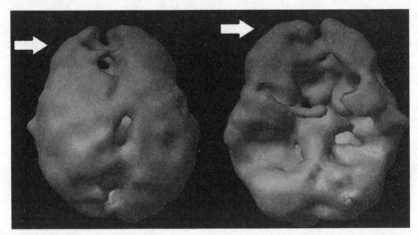

Top Down View   Underside View

Zackery's brain before HBOT.

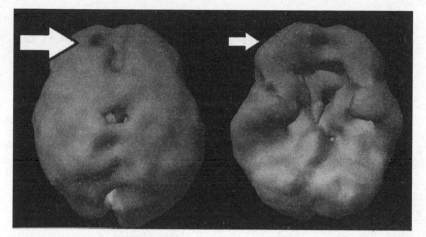

Top Down View   *Underside View*
Zackery's brain after HBOT.
Note the changes to the middle of the brain.

So what did Zack and his family notice after the HBOT sessions? On imaging, he had improvement in his prefrontal cortex and parietal lobe. This corresponded to his cognitive test scores showing improvements in his executive function and mathematical skills. His mother, Mercedes, reported that she thought he seemed more motivated to go to his numerous physical therapy appointments each week.

I salute this brave family and wish them the very best.

Current Research and TBI

So what does the research say about hyperbaric chamber therapy? The results are conflicting. The Cochrane Database, which is thought to be one of the most rigorous research libraries available, published a review in 2012 stating that for acute brain injury, mortality was decreased and the Glasgow

Coma Scale (GCS) was improved by 2.68 points on average. On the other hand, the research also showed that HBOT did not improve the overall recovery of the individuals and stated that many of these studies were poorly designed.[1]

There are more promising results for mild TBI when using HBOT, however. In 2013, a published study of fifty-six patients between one and five years post-TBI was conducted. They underwent forty one-hour sessions of HBOT at 1.5 atmospheres of pressure, which is less pressure than a diver would use for compression sickness and is equivalent to being about twelve feet under the ocean surface. Each patient in the study was struggling with some level of post-concussion syndrome.

After the series of forty sessions, the people in the study were reassessed by cognitive measures. Significant improvements were noted in quality of life and cognitive function based on cognitive computerized assessment and SPECT brain imaging.[2]

The research on HBOT for TBI is limited, however, and there are strong believers in both camps: those who have seen substantial benefits and those who have not. Certainly, there have been a number of highly successful cases, but there are also those who have seen little improvement. Because of the high investment of money and time to use a hyperbaric chamber (the cost is typically $100 to $200 per hour), this form of therapy is something I recommend as a second line of treatment, unless there are means or the situation is desperate. If the initial approaches to treating a TBI are ineffective, then I do suggest giving a trial of forty hours in the chamber.

There are hard- and soft-shell chambers, and both seem to work. Some study results suggest that a hard-shell chamber is far superior to the soft-shell inflatable chamber, but there is research as well as many personal experience reports testifying to the efficacy of the soft shell. The research clearly supports the use of a soft-shell chamber in a number of studies for TBI, which is why I recommend them, especially because of their ease of use since these chambers can be rented and used in the home. This cuts the cost of HBOT therapy considerably since one doesn't have to go to a clinic.

The soft-shell chamber is limited in the level of pressure that can be sustained for a treatment, however. Hard-shell chambers can go much higher as far as pressure, and some patients may benefit from these higher pressures. But I have found the lower pressures to be effective for most patients. The studies even show that the pressure is the most important part, because just breathing room air while in the chamber versus 100 percent oxygen still works. This is because the pressure driving the oxygen to the deeper structures is what is the key.

Two questions need to be asked:

- When is HBOT most useful?
- When is HBOT not useful at all?

I feel that HBOT can be most useful for those who've tried other therapies and haven't seen much improvement. Delivering oxygen at pressure to the deep nonhealing brain structures makes sense as a useful therapy, which is why I believe it can benefit many, especially those who suffered TBIs decades ago.

"Broadway Joe" Namath was a famous quarterback for the New York Jets football team back in the sixties. When he turned seventy-two years old, he began to have significant memory problems and struggled with depression. He had been knocked unconscious at least five times while he was playing, plus he was on the receiving end of countless other sub-concussive hits to the head.

Joe underwent 120 one-hour hyperbaric oxygen sessions and received significant improvements in both mood and cognitive function. What this says to me is that treatment many years later can help tremendously, but that treatment may involve many more sessions than forty. Still, I think that forty is a good number for most people.

A Closing Thought

Most cases of TBI are mild, but many people do not recover fully and consequently suffer chronic neurocognitive impairments. There is hope that some of the symptoms of chronic brain injury such as dizziness, poor focus, memory deficits, personality changes, irritability, and depression may be modified and improved through HBOT or other treatments. While the cost and time commitment are high, I do think hyperbaric chamber sessions should be considered after more accessible treatments, such as diet, nutrition, and brain training, have failed. HBOT can be life-changing. If you need a boost to help with your healing, whether you are early or late in the process, you owe it to yourself to look into how HBOT can help you.

Notes

1. McDonagh M, Helfand M, Carson S et al. Hyperbaric oxygen therapy for traumatic brain injury: a systematic review of the evidence. *Arch Phys Med Rehabil.* 2004;85(7):1198–204.

2. Boussi-Gross R, Golan H, Fishlev G et al. Hyperbaric oxygen therapy can improve post concussion syndrome years after mild traumatic brain injury - randomized prospective trial. *PLoS One.* 2013;8(11):e79995.

ACKNOWLEDGMENTS

'd first like to thank Dr. Daniel Amen for always inspiring me through his own passion for brain health and helping others. I'd like to thank my colleagues and friends for their support and guidance through this process. I'd like to thank my editors Mike Yorkey and Denise Silvestro for helping me bring this book to the "next level" and making it more accessible to readers.

And finally, I'd like to dedicate this book to public transportation and specifically Bus Route 532, without which I would not have had the dedicated time each day to write this book.

INDEX